Somatic Ego State Therapy for Trauma Healing

This book integrates Ego State therapy with body-based therapies to present a multidimensional approach to working with clients who have experienced trauma.

Drawing upon a range of important modalities, including Somatic Experiencing®, Polyvagal theory, Hypnotherapy, and Ego State therapy, Silvia Zanotta lays out a practical view of what it means to navigate the internal and external world in the aftermath of trauma. She provides an up-to-date applications-oriented view that prepares the practitioner to move beyond a one-size-fits-all treatment formula to meet the complexity of human experience. This approach holds that issues such as resistance, guilt and shame, rejection, and rage should be anticipated as a part of, more than an obstacle to, PTSD treatment. Case vignettes, transcript content, and step-by-step instructions for specific interventions and activities take the content of the chapters from theory to practice.

This is a practical, experiential book that will appeal to all professionals working with trauma, including psychotherapists, counsellors, body workers, and social workers.

Dr. Silvia Zanotta works as a psychologist and psychotherapist for children, adolescents, adults and families in private practice in Zurich, Switzerland. Before self-employment, she gained experience as a school- and educational psychologist and in child and adolescent psychiatry. She is a certified trainer and supervisor in Ego State Therapy International and Resource Therapy International as well as in Somatic Ego State Therapy, supervisor in hypnosis, as well as founder and co-chair of Ego State Therapy Switzerland.

Silvia Zanotta has been certified in Person-Centered-Therapy (Carl Rogers), Trauma-Therapy (PITT), Clinical Hypnosis (MEG and Ghyps), Ego State Therapy (FEST and ESTI) Resource Therapy, Somatic Experiencing® (SE Practitioner), and Somatic Ego State Therapy, including Energy Psychology in her work. She specializes in the treatment of traumatic stress, anxiety, phobia, OCD, autism, and somatic symptoms combining Ego State Therapy and hypnosis with somatic approaches. Dr. Zanotta, lecturer at the University of Applied Psychology in Zurich, has presented at major national and international conferences in Europe, Canada, and South Africa, she teaches in several European countries and has written various articles/publications on trauma and Ego State Therapy. This book was originally published in German by Auer in 2018 in Germany ("Wieder ganz werden. Traumaheilung mit Ego-State-Therapie und Körperwissen") and had to be reprinted within three months. A second edition followed in summer 2019, the third in summer 2022, and a fourth in 2023.

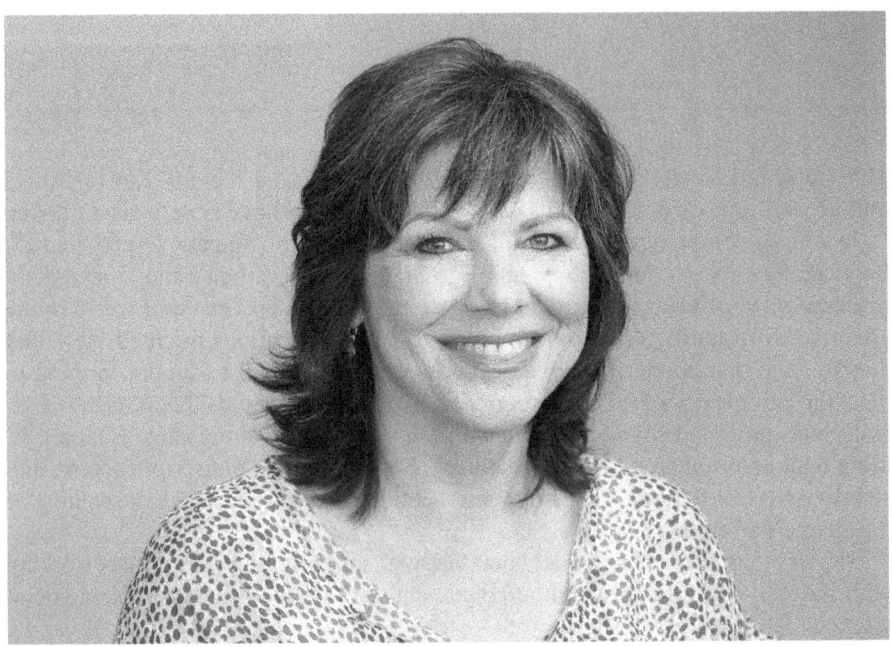

Photo by Corinne Koch

"In *Whole Again*, Silvia Zanotta, brilliantly integrates Ego State therapy with body-based therapies. The product is a model that effectively promotes a co-regulatory journey of healing in which the therapist guides the client through a process of re-embodiment in which safety is now experienced in both bodily feelings and thoughts."

Stephen W. Porges, author of *The Polyvagal Theory: Neurophysiological Foundations of Emotions, Attachment, Communication, and Self-regulation* and *The Pocket Guide to the Polyvagal Theory: The Transformative Power of Feeling Safe.*

"In this carefully thought-out application of Ego states, Silvia Zanotta demonstrates the importance of understanding how these states are anchored in our bodies. Using insights from Somatic Experiencing® and other body approaches, she shows how we can move from fragmentation to Wholeness."

Peter A Levine, Founder of Somatic Experiencing®, Author of *Waking the Tiger* and *An Autobiography: A Healing Journey.*

"I highly recommend this book to readers who are experienced in studying and practicing ego-state approaches, as well as to those who want to begin learning about this dynamic, highly effective path to healing posttraumatic difficulties. And while you are learning as you read the pages of this book, you will deeply appreciate the author's masterful clinical skills as well as her ability to take you on a deeply enriching journey toward self-empowerment and wholeness. Please welcome this rewarding new book into your library and into the heart of your clinical practice."

Maggie Phillips, author of *Reversing Chronic Pain*, of numerous papers and articles in the areas of Ego State therapy, hypnosis, Somatic Experiencing®, and the treatment of posttraumatic conditions and pain.

Somatic Ego State Therapy for Trauma Healing

Whole Again

Silvia Zanotta

Original book title: *Wieder ganz werden. Traumaheilung mit Ego-State-Therapie und Körperwissen.*
Translation from German into English: Tina Lüscher
Editorial Support: Suzi Tucker
Illustrations: Karin Hutter
Front Cover: From broken to beautiful: **Kintsugi** or **Kintsukuroi**, literally golden ("kin") and repair ("tsugi") is the Japanese art and philosophy (*wabi-sabi*) of repairing ceramics traditionally with lacquer and gold, leaving a gold seam where the cracks were and making it not only whole again, but more precious.

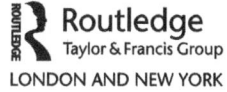

Routledge
Taylor & Francis Group
LONDON AND NEW YORK

Designed cover image: © Karin Hutter

First English edition published 2024
by Routledge
4 Park Square, Milton Park, Abingdon, Oxon OX14 4RN

and by Routledge
605 Third Avenue, New York, NY 10158

*Routledge is an imprint of the Taylor & Francis Group, an informa
business*

First German edition published by Auer, Heidelberg 2018

British Library Cataloguing-in-Publication Data
A catalogue record for this book is available from the British
Library

ISBN: 978-1-032-60814-3 (hbk)
ISBN: 978-1-032-60810-5 (pbk)
ISBN: 978-1-003-46060-2 (ebk)

DOI: 10.4324/9781003460602

Typeset in Times New Roman
by Apex CoVantage, LLC

Dedication

Dedicated with gratitude to my mentor Maggie Phillips, the consummate integrator and pioneer in combining hypnosis, Ego State therapy, and body approaches.

Contents

List of Figures

Foreword

By Maggie Phillips

My friendship with Silvia Zanotta began years ago when I accepted her invitation to teach a workshop on Ego State therapy in Zurich, where she lives. I sensed even in those early days when she was an organizer and student that she would make an excellent Ego State therapist because of her ability to connect with and draw out every person in the room, while engaging the entire group in supportive community. She was naturally demonstrating the two-fold process at the heart of the Ego State therapy approach.

Dr. Zanotta is a gifted, deeply caring, wise human being. Most impressive to me are her many ways of helping her clients to feel safe and cared about. My first book, *Healing the Divided Self* (Phillips & Frederick, 1995), emphasized the importance of safety, stability, and strengthening as the first stage of the transformational healing of traumatic experiences. This perspective on safety was expanded later on with Claire Frederick when we explored *conflict-free experience*, a resource already available to the self, which could be used for more rapid stabilization of safety for many clients.

My early work was an extension of the theory and practice generated by our teachers, John and Helen Watkins, who were co-creators of Ego State therapy (Watkins & Watkins, 1997). From the time of its origins, the model of Ego State therapy has been extremely popular in the hypnosis community, since that was the theoretical basis for the Watkins in understanding and working with states of the self that were linked to *fragmentation*, the dissociative splitting of self that occurs as an automatic response to trauma. From this orientation, hypnosis is used to explore, contain, and integrate fragmentation. More recent efforts have expanded Ego State methodology to include multi-modal methods such as those contained in this book.

Stephen Porges, whose seminal work on Polyvagal Theory has revolutionized the practice of trauma therapy through a new understanding of how the nervous system works, now insists that safety is *the* treatment for trauma. And safety, achieved through embodied attention to internal and external relational dimensions, is indeed the cornerstone of the approach presented in Dr. Zanotta's current book.

Although most trauma therapists agree that safety is essential, many therapists as well as their clients do not understand what safety actually entails. In *The Pocket*

Guide to the Polyvagal Theory: The Transformative Power of Feeling Safe Porges points out that the concepts we have of safety might not be in alignment with our body's sense of safety. In fact, he believes that safety is very different when defined by body responses versus cognitive ones (Porges, 2017). In other words, our left-brain evaluations of danger play a secondary role to our visceral reactions to people and places.

Also, Bessel van der Kolk (2014) has indicated that, if not repaired or released, trauma provokes collapse and fragmentation. He observes that fragmentation is part of the organism's attempt to maintain integrity in the face of overwhelming stress by splitting off intolerable aspects of self from the central self – physically, emotionally, mentally, and through the senses. This is the same splitting-off process explored by the Watkins' through uses of hypnosis in their Ego State model years before, although van der Kolk places more emphasis on working through the body.

Trauma therapy has only recently caught up with the interpersonal neurobiological approach, adding attachment theory in alignment with the social engagement ventral vagal circuit contributed by Porges, to provide a more psychobiological understanding of how strong relational experiences are essential to creating safety through the process of mutual co-regulation.

Somatic Ego State Therapy for Trauma Healing: Whole Again provides an essential perspective on how fundamental and essential elements of safety can be put into practice by stimulating and expanding somatic and relational pathways to heal a wide range of posttraumatic difficulties. Simply stated, this book teaches the reader in practical ways how to transform trauma by creating new relational and body experiences.

Dr. Zanotta sets the stage in her Introduction when she discusses psychotherapy as attachment and how corrective attachment experiences can occur through Ego State therapy with its focus both on relationship between client and therapist and on inner relationships among Ego State parts of the self.

The book unfolds with a beginning emphasis on how Ego State therapy can and should involve the body, helping clients shift from immobility to aliveness while creating new connections in brain function and attachment experience. Although somatic focus has become more pervasive in recent years (as evidenced by emphasis on the body by van der Kolk and others), what is exceptional about *Somatic Ego State Therapy for Trauma Healing: Whole Again* is the understanding that if the body is not included in the process of finding and working with ego states, as well as with the whole personality, transformation will be much slower and less complete, if it is possible at all.

In my own current methods, I combine Somatic Experiencing®, one of the earliest somatic approaches, which was developed by Dr. Peter Levine to treat trauma effectively, and Ego State therapy into an approach known as *Somatic Ego State Therapy*. The approach holds that very early developmental trauma, encoded only as implicit, preverbal memory, can be accessed and resolved with this method, as can other types of traumas that occur throughout the life span.

Dr. Zanotta skillfully interweaves a somatic thread into cases, illustrating the advantages of Ego State therapy in treating dissociation and freezing, anger and fear, pain and somatic symptoms, and she provides unique perspectives on shame as "the hidden emotion." Brief case examples appear throughout the book, providing the reader with rich models of how Ego State therapy can create change. Included as well are several detailed case presentations, including work with the four-year-old and infant ego states of a highly anxious university teacher, and multimodal Ego State therapy with a patient who suffered from severe trigeminal pain.

At the end of the book is an excellent section on "Practice Applications in Therapy." Methods are drawn from Ericksonian and clinical hypnosis, Somatic Experiencing®, Energy Psychology, and breathing and mindfulness. This feature alone is worth purchasing the book, providing many valuable tools for any therapist's toolbox.

I highly recommend *Somatic Ego State Therapy for Trauma Healing: Whole Again* to readers who are experienced in studying and practicing Ego state approaches, as well as to those who want to begin learning about this dynamic, highly effective path to healing posttraumatic difficulties. And while you are learning as you read the pages of this book, you will deeply appreciate the author's masterful clinical skills as well as her ability to take you on a deeply enriching journey toward self-empowerment and wholeness. Please welcome this rewarding new book into your library and into the heart of your clinical practice.

Maggie Phillips, PhD[1].

Maggie Phillips, author of numerous papers and articles in the areas of Ego State therapy, hypnosis, Somatic Experiencing®, and the treatment of posttraumatic conditions and pain, co-author of *Healing the Divided Self* and author of *Finding the Energy to Heal, Reversing Chronic Pain,* and *Freedom from Pain* co-authored with Peter Levine, was a pioneer in combining psychotherapeutic and somatic approaches.

Note

1 Dr. Phillips was Author/Coauthor of *Healing the Divided Self; Finding the Energy to Heal; Reversing Chronic Pain; Freedom from Pain; Empowering the Self through Ego-State Therapy; How to Create Lasting Change in Body Experience; Freedom from Pain: Guided Practices to Overcome Physical Pain; Meditation for Pain Relief.*

Reference

Phillips, M., & Frederick, C. (1995): *Healing the divided self: Clinical and Ericksonian hypnotherapy for dissociative conditions.* New York: Norton.

Preface

By Dr. Woltemade Hartman

To write the preface to this book written by my friend and colleague Dr. Silvia Zanotta, is indeed a great pleasure and an immense honor. It is a book about life and the immense impact trauma could have on all of us. This book cultivates not only a reawakening of what is meant by "being in flow and whole again." but also an understanding of the interdependence of us as humans on each other in our yearning for attachment, love, affection, and safety.

I had the privilege of working therapeutically with Dr. Zanotta during a psychotherapy congress in Kathmandu, Nepal in 2008. At that time, I had taught a workshop on grief and bereavement and Dr Zanotta graciously availed herself for a demonstration regarding some personal loss. To my knowledge, this was her first personal mind-body-experience with Ego State therapy as we know it today. Since that session, Dr. Zanotta has been on a personal and professional journey expanding her knowledge, wealth of experience, and clinical applications of Ego State therapy and body work. However, at some stage, both she and I expressed a need for more knowledge regarding the role of the body and "body wisdom" in psychotherapy, as well as the somatic and neurophysiological foundations of so-called "parts of the personality" or "ego states." This quest for wisdom prompted us to join the Somatic Experiencing® training of Dr. Peter Levine presented by Dr. Maggie Phillips and Dr. Sonia Gomes in South Africa. The result was a sustained tour de force of collaborative effort to learn and discover the intricate relationship between Ego State therapy combined with the Polyvagal Theory of Dr. Stephen Porges and the Somatic Experiencing® techniques of Dr. Peter Levine.

Ego State therapy was the creation of Dr. John and Helen Watkins from the United States. The Watkins' did not conceptualize the ego as one monolithic entity, as Freud did, but rather as consisting of parts, or ego states. They conceptualized an ego state as an organized system of behaviour and experience whose elements are bound together by some common principle, which is separated from other such states by a boundary that is permeable (Watkins & Watkins, 1997). Their theory was based on the original work of Paul Federn, a close associate and colleague of Freud. Federn conceptualised ego states as shifting energies within the personality. John and Helen Watkins formulated a theory and treatment model for what became known as Ego State therapy. The original theory of ego states and Ego State therapy as defined and described by the Watkins (1997), was progressively becoming outdated and in urgent need of revision and redefinition to also include the neurophysiological foundations of ego states and its connection to interpersonal neurobiology. As such, I redefined ego states as "neuro-physiological and psychological manifestations of the autonomic nervous system response which may develop as a reaction to certain life experiences, both positive and negative" (Hartman, 2018). However, in this book Dr. Zanotta takes this definition of ego states and Ego State therapy a step further. She integrates and uniquely combines disparate psychotherapeutic and psychobiological approaches such as neuroscience, psychotherapy, body work, interpersonal neurobiology and Ego State therapy into an integrated approach which Dr. Maggie Phillips and she refer to as "Somatic Ego State Therapy."

It is a known fact that psychological trauma may fragment the mind. However, in this book we discover that trauma has a major impact on both mind and body. We learn that our minds desperately try to leave traumatic experiences behind us through internal psychological fragmentation, but at the same time, our bodies cling to the memories and stay trapped in the past. Dr. Zanotta vividly describes and illustrates how "split off" or dissociated ego states that remain frozen in time, moment and context, can become "unstuck" again by resetting the autonomic nervous system response and thereby reestablishing a sense of safety, wholeness, flow, coherence, connectedness with others, self-regulation, and embodiment. She elaborates on how clients can get stuck in experiences of threat, dread, mental and physical trauma, and a kind of paralyzing shutdown and collapse. Shame, guilt, anger, chronic pain, major depression, and self-loathing may follow in the wake of such imposed helplessness and despair. She then continues to describe in detail how to "unfreeze" such states and suggests various practical techniques to guide and facilitate a process of reintegrating such dissociated ego states and how to reestablish wholeness, flow, containment, and self-regulation. Dr. Zanotta also provides us with a detailed description of an array of useful intervention strategies and how to practically implement a somatic approach to Ego State therapy in alleviating the debilitating effects of traumatic stress and posttraumatic stress disorders. The book is replete with various case vignettes and substantiated with evidence-based and well-designed research.

Dr. Zanotta's inspiring vision and wealth of wisdom and experience becomes clear in her book and is quite remarkable. This book is essential reading material for both beginners and more experienced practitioners of parts work, Polyvagal Theory, Somatic Experiencing®, and bodywork in general. I have no doubt that Dr. Zanotta, with this book, has now secured her position not only in the forefront of trauma theorists, but also as practitioner and as teacher. All of us in the therapeutic and neuroscience community, psychologists, psychotherapists, clinicians, and professionals in the medical fraternity alike, can only benefit from this inspirational journey to learn about the fascinating world of ego states, its connection to trauma, and how to become unstuck and whole again. I am quite sure the book will become a classic in "parts work," Ego State therapy, and for body therapy.

Woltemade Hartman, Ph.D. from South Africa was a student of the Watkins' and brought Ego State therapy to Europe, Australia, and to many Asian countries. He teaches Ego State therapy all over the world.

Clinical and Educational Psychologist, and Psychotherapist
Director of the Milton. H. Erickson Institute of South Africa (MEISA)
Founding and Past-President of Ego State Therapy International (ESTI)
Executive Board member of the International Society of Hypnosis (ISH)

Introduction

A Prismatic View of Trauma Treatment

The Body Knows the Way

Trauma sufferers, in their healing journeys, learn to dissolve their rigid defenses. In this surrender they move from frozen fixity to gently thawing and, finally, free flow. In healing the divided self from its habitual mode of dissociation, they move from fragmentation to wholeness. In becoming embodied they return from their long exile. They come home to their bodies and know embodied life, as though for the first time. While trauma is hell on earth, its resolution may be a gift from the gods.

(Levine, 2010, p. 356)

In working with people as a psychotherapist, supervisor, and trainer, it has been my experience that psychotherapeutic techniques alone do not account for a successful therapy. There are two essential factors that are just as important for emotional and mental healing: *Relationship building* and *body experience*.

My therapeutic work is based on the following principles:

a) The implicit solution of symptoms in the unconscious (Milton Erickson)
b) The actualizing tendency in the therapeutic context of unconditional acceptance (Carl Rogers)
c) The holistic mindful experience in a safe relationship via Focusing (Eugene Gendlin)
d) The model of parts in Ego State therapy (John and Helen Watkins)
e) The possibility of trauma resolution on a physical level with Somatic Experiencing® (Peter Levine), and the combination of d) and e), respectively: Somatic Ego State Therapy (Maggie Phillips).

Since every person is unique in their combination of personality parts, it is only logical to keep re-attuning to every client and to their individual needs and distinct actualizing tendency: Every human deserves a bespoke treatment. I act on the assumption that there is an ancient wisdom of self-healing inherent in every human organism. If this "inner wisdom," embodied in *body knowledge*, is included in therapy, many problems and symptoms can be solved more easily.

DOI: 10.4324/9781003460602-1

Nearly 25 years ago, when, for the very first time, I was facing a client with complex trauma who obviously felt threatened by me, despite my friendly attempts to build a relationship, and was constantly on the verge of dissociating, making me feel just as helpless and powerless in my desperate attempt to offer a safe setting, I understood how important building relationships and safety are for successful psychotherapy. Thanks to my supervisor's close monitoring and a training in psycho-imaginative trauma therapy with Luise Reddemann, I was able to reach this client, as her window of tolerance (Siegel, 1999) slowly started increasing. My curiosity having been sparked, I wanted to know more about the effects of trauma on body and soul, and to gain a better understanding of psycho-physiological, intra- and interpsychic processes. I pursued trainings in clinical hypnosis, Ego State therapy, and Somatic Experiencing® trauma therapy soon after. I became deeply involved with Ego State therapy and body experience so that I was able to offer people with complex trauma a safe therapeutic space in which they could find hope for control and stability, and where change towards healing became possible. Since traumatic experiences are always stored in the somatic memory, it is essential to include the body when applying Ego State therapy.

Thanks to hypno-somatic, multimodal Ego State therapy or *Somatic Ego State Therapy* – the combination of Ego State therapy with body procedures created and taught by Maggie Phillips – psychotherapists can use the body as a resource. Though always available as a useful resource, many psychotherapists lack the tools to enlist the body during therapy. By including the body, the clients not only learn to better self-regulate but can also access unconscious or preverbal trauma stored in the implicit body memory, as well as somatic ego states. For that to happen, a safe therapeutic relationship and appropriate timing and pacing following the rhythm of the client are necessary.

In the course of my psychotherapeutic work, I have experienced repeatedly how important it is to include body signals as a resource. This is true for me in my role as a therapist – how I deal with my reactions to the client and with my own body sensations – and it is true for the clients whose bodies often present the solution if the therapist is open for it.

> *I feel so much better. I feel much stronger, less upset by my mother's phone calls. After every therapy session, I am amazed that the session is so helpful, and I am so grateful.*
>
> (46-year-old client after working with boundaries and changing position, cf. Chapter 8, the exercise "Restoring Boundaries")

> *I have more space in my body now. My shoulders are more open, something is shifting. I am allowed to take my space . . . The final image is beautiful and sensual. The body process has deeply touched me. Finally, I was able to defend myself!*
>
> (40-year-old client)

Thanks to Ego State therapy, painful states from childhood could be influenced in a soothing way, so that I felt warmth and positive feelings. By anchoring these positive feelings in my body, I can still access them later, when I need them.
(53-year-old client)

Focusing on somatic sensations and reactions has raised my awareness of the slightest changes and signs in the face and body of the person in front of me. To me, change is only possible when a client can experience and understand in an integrated way. When clients have a new experience or feel a change, it shows immediately in their body sensations. Clients then report shifts such as: "Something is starting to release." "It's relaxing." "Now it is quiet." "It feels lighter."

When working psychotherapeutically with people affected by trauma, you often find attachment issues besides dissociative phenomena. These issues strongly influence the building of relationships and the psychotherapeutic process. Early bonding experiences are delicate. They depend on a fine interaction between the attachment figure and the infant, whose needs should be recognized and responded to in a sensitive way so that the child can bond safely during the first few years. This bonding is the foundation for the psychological wellbeing and trust in other people. It is critical for the psychological health of a person and for building relationships. According to Guy Bodenmann, psychology professor and leading attachment figure from Zürich, about half of the children in Switzerland develop an insecure attachment pattern. His 2017 newspaper article shows how relevant this issue is regarding the care-taking model of infants during their first three years.[1]

According to Frederick (2012), some sort of inner attachment representation occurs in children at the age of two, meaning an inner map of neural networkings of sorts in the brain, which from now on influence self-regulation, self-perception, and the behavior of the individual. This attachment pattern seems to be not only the most important imprint for affect- and self-regulation (Schore, 2003), but also for the further development of the brain (Frederick 2012). An insecure inner attachment representation, early attachment disorders, are the direct cause of complex posttraumatic stress disorders and of dissociation. If, during the development, there are further traumatic experiences, the psychopathology is reinforced. Many psychotherapeutic attempts to create a safe attachment either have not proven successful or they involve a prolonged course of therapy. By nourishing and strengthening the self and the whole personality, and also by creating safe attachments with resourceful ego states or with "ideal parents," on an inner stage, Ego State therapy opens up the possibility of changing the connections formed in the brain at the age of two in a sustained way towards stabilization, self-regulation, and improvement of self-esteem. This also has an effect on the behavior and the interpersonal relationships on the outer stage. Moreover, the human organism possesses a rich potential for self-healing powers which can be stimulated not only on a psychological, but also on a physical level, and can bring surprising solutions, along the lines of hypnotherapy. By contacting preverbal ego states, manifesting on the somatic level in a diffuse way, the combination with body psychotherapeutic approaches such as Somatic Experiencing®, trauma therapy not only facilitates the dissolution of a freeze response and of dissociation but also the healing of pre-, peri-, and postnatal traumas.

In the first chapter of this book, "Hypnosomatic Ego State therapy," I present a synthesis of Ego State therapy and hypnosis as well as body-oriented psychotherapy, based on current neurobiological (Porges, 2009, 2022) and psychological findings. With a stable and clearly structured relationship between the client and the therapist as a solid base, including the body can be crucial for the success of psychotherapy, especially with unconscious and dissociated preverbal traumatization or attachment ruptures that are stored in the body memory.

In the second chapter, important principles of Ego State therapy are highlighted: Dealing with resistance and blockages, with ego states that act in a destructive way and are at the core of Ego State therapy, and the many facets of corrective relational experiences on the inner stage. These are advanced issues of Ego State therapy that can be challenging for therapists because of their complexity.

In the majority of chapters, I detail my inclusive approach, showing well-tested techniques regarding the specific challenges in the treatment of traumatized people. Case studies help demonstrate and clarify various ways to apply this integrative perspective. I not only deal with phenomena such as preverbal trauma, dissociation, pain, anxiety, and anger, I also highlight the essential aspects of restoring and respecting boundaries. I have paid special attention to the issue of shame and its treatment. Interestingly, there is little literature on this hidden and often unrecognized emotion, yet it is ever-present in the treatment of trauma. I have integrated the therapeutic approach to shame recommended by Peter Levine into my work. In Chapter 6, this highly effective procedure is presented and illustrated with descriptions of actual processes.

In the final chapter, I provide practical instructions, exercises, and interventions.

Psychotherapy as an Attachment Workshop

Efficacy studies suggest that the quality of therapeutic relationship building is an important prerequisite for the success of a therapy, including the adequate treatment of complaints (Miller, S. 2018, https://youtu.be/6OJur59U0jY).

When two people meet and interact, their bodies automatically engage in a psychophysiological interaction, their rhythms attuning to each other (Feldman, 2017). The quality arising from this synchronization is also called *attunement*. This ability for rhythmic attunement with a close attachment figure is the foundation for learning to regulate emotional states (Trevarthen, 1999). Gestures and facial expressions, as well as hormonal processes and autonomous activities in the nervous system and brain of both people adapt to one another. However, dysregulated behavior has an alienating effect on relationships and compromises the ability to recover and develop resilience (van der Kolk, 2010). A child experiencing a lack of attunement with their attachment figure is in a state of over excitement and cannot react adequately to stresses and strains. Because the child cannot emotionally regulate, the probability increases that they will react habitually with fight or flight (Scaer, 2005).

These congruencies in the nonverbal behavior between mother and child play a vital role in the development of safe attachment. Physiological synchronization is associated with phases of mutually experienced positive attunement (Feldman, 2007; Woltering et al., 2015). For this reason, the concept of "repair" (Tronick, 1989) is vital, representing the ability of an attachment dyad to transform errors and conflicted interactions into communication and behavior patterns and thus to restore harmony. When there is a safe attachment between two people, even ruptures do not portend disruption or pathology. Children having experienced many "repairs" during their development exhibit high self-efficacy and the expectation of being able to effectively repair "injured attachments" with primary attachment figures. These children can cope with external stressors and remain socially engaged in phases of interpersonal tension. This ability to stay attuned in dyadic interactions even when things become stressful is accompanied by effective self-regulation (Feldman, Greenbaum, & Yirmiya, 1999). Thus, being able to *repair attachments* and to make peace requires emotional *self-regulation* and vice-versa. In terms of a circular process, solidarity in relationships is consolidated, creating safe attachments. Safe attachment experiences manifest throughout the whole body because they have a deep effect on physical, emotional, and mental wellbeing. Neurobiological attachment research has borne this idea out (i.e., Feldman, 2017, 2012; Porges, 2017).

These findings regarding attachment may also be interesting for the dyadic working relationship in psychotherapy. For therapeutic interventions to be well accepted, the relational level must be established and clarified first. For people who find it difficult to trust due to earlier trauma, it is healing to keep experiencing that despite interruptions the human connection in a therapeutic relationship can persist or be re-established. The therapist's resonance helps such clients to experience being seen, heard, appreciated and understood, sometimes for the very first time.

Keep in mind, resonance is more than empathy. Resonance is where we experience relation/connection with our client on an energy level without losing ourselves.

(Paulsen, 2009, p. 85)

When conscious or unconscious memories of violating or traumatic experiences in interpersonal relationships are awakened in the client during the interaction with the therapist, the autonomic nervous system reacts immediately. The environment and the person vis-à-vis, or one's own overwhelming affects or body, are experienced as dangerous rather than as safe, triggering a cascade of defense mechanisms. These processes tend to remain unconscious. Stephen Porges calls this involuntary system of perception seeking safety, *neuroception*. As soon as neuroception signals danger, the body physiology changes abruptly. This occurs not only for the client but sometimes for the therapist. The traumatic experience of the client is actualized in the here and now of the therapeutic interaction and *in the client's* body. The threat can also be felt physically by the therapist via their neuroception, who now also assesses the environment or their own aroused autonomic processes as being dangerous. Feelings of countertransference arise. Therefore, it is most important that therapists learn to self-regulate in their contacts with the clients because the inability to influence emotional states of arousal make it more difficult for clients to profit from therapy (Jaycox, Foa, & Morral, 1998). In his polyvagal theory, published 1995, Stephen Porges pointed out that acute stress visibly influences social behavior and is expressed first in the face and in the prosody of the voice.

Research investigating the change in the size of the pupil in a social context shows how extremely fast and unconsciously these neuroception processes happen. In one study, a group of men were shown portraits of women, and they were asked to rank the women according to their attractiveness. Half the women pictured in the portraits had received eye drops enlarging their pupils before the photoshoot. Nearly all of the men rated the women with enlarged pupils as more attractive, without being aware of the difference (Hess, 1975). Later, imaging methods showed that eyes with larger pupils caused a stronger activation of the amygdala in the brain of the viewer of the portraits, irrespective of how the attractiveness of the person was rated (Demos et al., 2008). Kret (2017) suggested that infants unconsciously imitate the size of the pupils of the eyes facing them, and showed that, through social learning, larger pupils can be associated with love, care, and interest on the part of those who are with them.

Larger pupils make the vis-à-vis seem more likable, but only if one's own pupils also dilate. Moreover, the involuntary imitation of the pupil's size seems to be a precondition for empathy. When seeing sad faces with smaller pupils, the pupils of the test subjects also contracted (Harrison et al., 2006).

When, in the course of a psychotherapeutic interaction, a regressive state emerges in the client so that an injured or protective ego state manifests in the client's conscious, there can be ruptures in the contact that are more or less subtle, accompanied by defense mechanisms (Scaer, 2005). If such irritations are addressed in the here and now – responding also nonverbally to the client's nervous system longing for safety – the connection between client and therapist is deepened and trust is increased.

The process by which the nervous systems of the two people involved mutually affect each other, thus pendulating into an optimally balanced tone, is called *coregulation* (Levine, Porges, & Phillips, 2015). When the therapeutic relationship allows the client to have a corrective relational experience in which it is possible to "coregulate" in contact with the therapist, the probability of the client being able to regulate outside the sessions increases.

This development contributes indirectly to psychological stamina, for, the better the self-regulation, the more self-efficient people feel. They become more courageous and tend to face everyday challenges more readily. This enhances their feeling of being in control. With growing resilience, the window of tolerance for a greater range of arousal widens (Siegel, 2010), and, with that, the ability to tolerate and endure difficult feelings and still feel capable of acting. As a consequence, the client can now survive unsettling life events with relatively little damage and is able to recover.

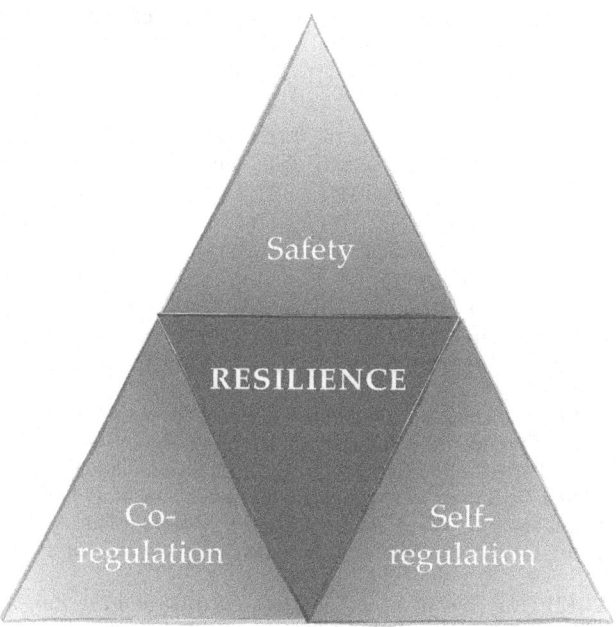

Figure 0.1 Safety and self-regulation facilitate resilience

Corrective Attachment Experiences with Ego State Therapy

Ego State therapy offers useful instruments for corrective experiences, facilitating not only new interpersonal but also intrapsychic relationship experiences – indirectly strengthening the ability to self-regulate. Clients not only learn to relate to their parts in a new way, but the parts can also engage in healthy relationships with each other, thus fostering integration and flexibility of the entire personality.

Here, therapists are role models. They exemplify how to deal respectfully with the clients and all their ego states and demonstrate how a safe relationship to the ego states and the clients can be built.

Ego State therapy offers manifold possibilities to make up for what was missed in childhood and youth, and to change or recreate what was missing in clients' development. New neural connections are created, which change thoughts, sensations, and behavior. For instance, attachment traumas can be healed by building alliances on the inner stage, providing safety and facilitating stability.

Since our organism is always searching for safety via neuroception, clients can only create these corrective experiences if they are supported *within the therapeutic relationship, through coregulation*, to regulate their nervous system, and be able to constantly improve their ability to self-regulate. This process by itself is a corrective experience. If clients can allow themselves to feel safe and to relax in their contact with the therapist, this experience can also have a positive effect on the relationships in their environment. A relaxed nervous system not only facilitates the ability to self-regulate but also fosters creative problem solving.

Note

1 Information given in an interview in the Tages-Anzeiger (Swiss local newspaper) on 24 October 2017: "Nearly every second child suffers from an attachment disorder – what forms of care can help in this case?"

References

Demos, K. E., Kelley, W. M., Ryan, S. L., Davis, F. C., & Whalen' P. J. (2008): Human Amygdala Sensitivity to the Pupil Size of Others. *Cortex, 18(12)*: 2729–2734.

Feldman, R. (2017): The Neurobiology of Human Attachments. *Trends in Cognitive Sciences, 21(2)*: 80–99.

Feldman, R. (2012): Bio-behavioral synchrony: A model for integrating biological and microsocial behavioral processes in the study of parenting. *Parenting, 12*: 154–164.

Feldman, R. (2007): Parent-infant Synchrony: Biological Foundations and Developmental Outcomes. *Current Directions in Psychological Science, 16(6)*: 340–345.

Feldman, R., Greenbaum, C. W., & Yirmiya (1999): Mother-infant Affect Synchrony as an Antecedent of the Emergence of Self-control. *Developmental Psychology, 35(1)*: 223–231.

Frederick, C. (2012): *The Evolution of Ego State Therapy into the Post-Modern World: Intersubjectivity, Countertransference Trances, Personal Mythology and Developmental Repair.* (Workshop in Zurich organized by Ego State Therapy Switzerland. 4–5 May 2012).

Harrison, N. A., Singer, T., Rothstein, P., Dolan, R. J., & Critchley, H. D. (2006): Pupillary Contagion: Central Mechanisms Engaged in Sadness Processing. *Scan I*, 5–17.

Hess, E. H. (1975): The Role of Pupil Size in Communication. *Scientific American, 233(5)*: 110–112, 116–119.

Jaycox, L. H., Foa, E. B., Morral, A. R. (1998): Influence of Emotional Engagement and Habituation on Exposure Therapy for PTSD. *Journal of Consulting and Clinical Psychology, 66(1)*: 185–192.

Kret, M. E. (2017): The role of pupil size in communication. Is there room for learning? *Cognition and Emotion, 94(2)*: 173–174.

Levine, P. (2010): *In an Unspoken Voice: How the Body Releases Trauma and Restores Goodness.* Berkeley, North Atlantic Books.

Levine, P., Porges, S. W., & Phillips, M. (2015): *Healing Trauma and Pain Through Polyvagal Science*: E-Book. www.maggiephillipsphd.com

Paulsen, S. (2009): *Looking through the Eyes of Trauma and Dissociation. An Illustrated Guide for EMDR Therapists and Clients.* BookSurge Publishing.

Porges, S. W. (2022): *Polyvagal Theory: A Science of Safety*. Frontiers (in Integrative Neuroscience) May 2022, Volume 16. Open Access: Front. Integr. Neurosci. 16:871227. doi. 10.3389/fnint.2022.871227

Porges, S. W. (2017): *Die Polyvagal-Theorie und die Suche nach Sicherheit*. Lichtenau/ Westfalen: G.P. Probst.

Porges, S. W. (2009): The Polyvagal Theory: New insights into adaptive reactions of the autonomic nervous system. *Cleveland Clinic Journal of Medicine, 76(2)*: 86–89.

Scaer, R. (2005): *The Trauma Spectrum: Hidden Wounds and Human Resiliency*. W.W. Norton & Co.

Schore, A. N. (2003): *Affect Dysregulation and Disorders of the Self*. New York: Norton.

Siegel, D. J. (2010): *The Mindful Therapist. A Clinician's Guide to Mindsight and Neural Integration*. Norton & Co.

Siegel, D. J. (1999): *The Developing Mind. Toward a Biology of Interpersonal Experience*. Gardners Books.

Trevarthen, C. (1999) in: Porges, S. W. (2010). *Die Polyvagal-Theorie. Neurophysiologische Grundlagen der Therapie. Emotionen, Bindung, Kommunikation und ihre Entstehung*. Paderborn: Junfermann.

Tronick, E. Z. (1989). Emotions and Emotional Communication in Infants. *American Psychologist, 44(2)*: 112.

van der Kolk, B. (2010) in: Porges, S. W. (2010). *Die Polyvagal-Theorie. Neurophysiologische Grundlagen in der Therapie. Emotionen, Bindung, Kommunikation und ihre Entstehung*. Parderborn: Junfermann.

Woltering, S., Lishyk, V., Elliott, B., Ferraro, L., & Granic, I. (2015): Dyadic Attunement and Physiological Synchrony During Mother-Child Interactions: An Exploratory Study in children With and Without Externalizing Behavior Problems. *Journal of Psychopathology and Behavioral Assessment, 37(4)*. doi: 10.1007(s10862-015-9480-3.

Chapter 1

Hypnosomatic Ego State Therapy

Ego State Therapy and the Body

Two introductory examples from my own work illustrate how helpful it can be to include the body in psychotherapy, and how Ego State therapy can be combined quite naturally with body approaches such as Somatic Experiencing® trauma therapy.

In our first meeting, a 52-year-old female client in a managerial capacity is on the verge of breaking down due to severe workplace bullying and constant overwork. She is suffering from intense fear. She reports severe emotional neglect and a lack of parental care in early childhood. In the first session, she is overwhelmed by her feelings of fear. The therapist asks for her permission to speak directly to the frightened ego state, a four-year-old girl who is all on her own. The therapist then explains to the little one that it is over, that now she has the power to change that memory and her immediate environment in a way that she feels good, safe, and cared for. The four-year-old girl settles in a meadow where the sun is shining, where she can run around lightheartedly, where a kind woman and a caring man play with her and give her safety, love, and appreciation. The therapist then invites her to create a safe boundary of glass around this safe meadow, and the client does so. The client settles and feels relieved.

As an additional stabilizing measure, to take distance from the overwhelming feelings, the therapist invites the client to meet her inner observer: "The fact that you can speak about your thoughts, feelings and body sensations shows that you can observe them. So, you are more than those fears. Imagine standing behind yourself, putting one hand on your shoulder and observing yourself acceptingly. Can you do that?" The client withdraws to the "position of an observer," calming down even more. The distance is good for her. The therapist continues: "Whenever it gets too

DOI: 10.4324/9781003460602-2

much, you can withdraw to that position of an observer and watch from a distance." After that, the client feels relieved, relaxed, and has a pleasant feeling in her chest.

In the second session, the four-year-old still feels safe and cared for in her meadow. However, the client is suffering from a terror, threatening to destabilize her. The therapist invites her to explore this fear and the body sensations associated with it. The client feels powerless, incapable of action. She is overcome by enormous fear, what she describes as "undefinable" and "unfathomable," a very small ego state, a baby alone in the cellar. She lacks the words, is completely helpless, caught up in these diffuse sensations. Since her level of arousal is very high and she no longer feels her body, the therapist asks for her permission to sit next to her and to touch her on her shoulder. At the same time, the therapist soothes the baby, also explaining to her: "This is not happening now. You are safe now. You are not alone. I am with you. It is over!" Her soothing voice gives the adult client (and her baby ego state, of course) containment, and she starts settling. Now and then the therapist lets her pause and asks about her body sensations: "What is it like now?" After a few minutes, the client starts feeling her body and her physical boundaries. The therapist asks: "Who could hold the baby and protect her? She is so terribly lonely!" With the support of the therapist, who is suggesting different possibilities of how to care for the baby, the client begins to describe a mother figure, first tentatively, then more and more accurately, who is relating to the baby 100 percent – nourishing, holding, protecting, and providing warmth, comfort, and safety. As the baby has everything she needs and has also understood that it will always be like that from now on, the therapist asks the client how she feels. Her sensation and state have completely changed. "Light, cheerful, strong, invulnerable" is how she describes how she feels. "Nothing can knock me over!" The therapist writes these sentences on a piece of paper, which she hands over to the client at the end of the session. The client, now completely in her adult state, cannot quite trust those new feelings and sensations yet. It is utterly understandable that she and the baby need time and continuity for this big change. The mother figure must keep proving and showing on the inner stage that she is there. The baby still needs to be greatly appreciated by the therapist for her profound suffering and for how terrible it was to be without body contact to the mother. The therapist assures the baby that she cannot be blamed, that that should not have happened and that, like every baby, she has a right to be loved and cared for. The therapist adds: "You are utterly lovable just the way you are. I am happy that at last you are safe, the way you always would have deserved it!" In the following session, the client reports being quasi "transformed" since last time.

At the end of the therapy, looking back at the whole therapeutic process, the client reports that the first two sessions had been very impressive. In the first session, the safety of the four-year-old girl in the meadow had already triggered physical changes. In the second session, she had come "back into her body," and this had happened through the touch on her shoulder. It had been an aha! moment: "Oh, yes, I am here!"

She also reports that her whole attitude towards life had changed through the therapy. Constantly moving back and forth between the present and early childhood (the ego states) had been "dramatic" for her. But now she had new strategies. The new inner images were helpful, she could evoke them any-time. Thus, "Fidgety Philipa" (a resource state that showed up in the course of the therapy) was consistently skipping in front of her. She was also feeling strong in real life.

This case shows how important a supportive therapeutic relationship is for self-soothing through coregulation, especially when the client is overwhelmed by younger or preverbal ego states and existential fear.

Coregulation happens here through being present, enduring, staying with it, *containment* (Bion, 1970). The psychoanalyst Wilfred Bion suggested a model for therapeutic interaction that leans on the mother-child relationship. According to this, coregulation happens through containment, just as a child projects over-whelming feelings onto the mother and can then understand and handle them. The mother reflects them back to the child in a way that allows the child to tol-erate their feelings. In hypnosomatic Ego State therapy, the existentially threat-ened ego states flooded with panic are accompanied in a soothing way, through a pleasant prosody of the voice and sometimes also with a few carefully applied physical touches, pausing and a mindful perception, so the client can realize that "it is over," and that they are now in a safe place and can build their inner environment according to their own wishes until they feel completely safe and protected. Bion (1970) suggested that a "triangulating place" in the therapist is needed for this process of containment, a so-called "thinking container" in which the therapist can process and interpret the material received, "predigest" it, be-fore reflecting it back to the client.

Hypnosomatic Ego State therapy takes this a step further. By emphasizing mind-ful sensory perception, an observer ego state, an "inner observer" – one who helps to create distance from intrusive overwhelming feelings – is activated in order to promote stability and autonomy in the client.

In the sessions that followed, the client was shown additional soothing breath-ing techniques and tapping techniques like EFT known in the US. For support and coregulation in her daily life, security-giving trances were offered, which were recorded on her mobile phone. She can listen to these recordings between ses-sions, which she feels is especially helpful given the difficult situations that she keeps having to face in everyday life. Thus, the client can constantly improve and increase her abilities to self-regulate and slowly find greater stability.

The Solution "Emerges"

With another excerpt, we want to show how a preverbal ego state can be helped to express on a body level through a somatic bridge, and how, via involuntary physical processes, a solution for an inner-psychic predicament can just "emerge." This requires that a safe therapeutic relationship has already been established and that there is permission to act out body impulses accurately, letting them happen while both client and therapist attend the process in a mindful and positively curious way.

The client, in her mid-40s, let us call her Ms. Y, wants to work on her extreme aversion to her mother. In fact, she wants to get rid of her sensations of disgust when she is with her mother. The therapist asks her to imagine a situation where she experienced disgust and to feel into it, and then to describe as accurately as possible what it is like for her. Client: "I feel like yelling. I bite my cheeks, everything is contracting, tensing up. I see my mother in the color of clay. I am about to throw up!" She starts to choke. Therapist: "Just stay with it and observe your body sensations . . . May I speak directly to this tensed up part?" The client gives permission. Therapist: "What shall I call you?" No answer. The client: "She is still very small." The therapist suggests: "Shall I call you 'Everything-is-contracting'?" The client nods. Therapist: "Everything-is-contracting, I have heard from Ms. Y. that you feel very much disgusted by your mother. Somehow, you feel threatened, she scares you." The client nods. Therapist: "Now listen carefully: This is not happening now. It is over. You are safe now. This is a memory stored in your brain and in your body. And you can now change that memory. You have the power and the right to change this memory until you feel completely comfortable. For instance, you can shrink your mother until she is the size of a pea, you can put her further away until she no longer disgusts you. Make her small and create distance!" Client: "I'm not able to think yet!" Therapist: "What does your body want? What do you feel?" The client's feet and hands twitch nearly imperceptibly. The therapist picks up on that: "Mind the smallest impulses, Everything-is-contracting, your body knows exactly what has to be done. Just let it happen, slowly, in slow motion. Let your body do what it has always wanted to do, but was not able to do then . . . What does your body want?" Client: "It wants to kick. But it doesn't dare to yet." Therapist: "Then imagine that it is kicking, in slow motion, very slowly, give yourself and your body all the time you need . . ." After a few minutes, the client's hands and feet start moving (her feet are on a cushion). The therapist goes to the client and holds the cushion so that the kicking feet now encounter resistance. Therapist: "Very good. Slowly. Give your body time to release. Slowly, so that you can always feel what it is like. Very good. That's it!" The client starts struggling using her hands and feet, first tentatively, then more and more clearly and strongly, a defensive struggling in slow motion. The therapist offers resistance at the feet, supporting and slowing things down by saying: "Very slowly, very good, even slower." When the client's breathing stops: "And – breathe! Just keep breathing easily! That's it! And now feel again what it feels like now!" The therapist can feel that a lot of energy and strength are released. She invites the client to pause, now and again, to track what she is feeling. Therapist: "Only you know for how long your body has to repeat that, how long it takes until it is okay." When being asked during one of the pauses, what it is like, the client answers: "I feel like a beetle on its back, but I have a lot of strength. There is a golden egg around me protecting me, a safe boundary for me, my back is connected to the egg, I am like a scarab. I can defend myself. At last I am protected and free." Therapist: "Does the name 'Everything-is-contracting' still fit now?" The client's answer is no. Therapist: "What can I call you?" Client: "Golden Beetle." Therapist: "Do you need anything else, Golden Beetle?" After the client has said no, the therapist addresses the adult client of today: "What is it like now, Ms. Y.? Client: "I am still in the feeling of gold. It is very pleasant." The therapist asks her to go back and feel into the situation at the beginning of the session, when she was feeling so much disgust towards her mother. Therapist: "How is it now?" Client: "Everything is much farther away."

When the client puts herself in the "situation of disgust," her body reacts immediately and very violently. She "feels like screaming," the baby's scream of protest; "biting," an early defense reaction; "everything is contracting," her body assumes a position of protection or, more accurately, freezes, also a defense reaction, in service of her self-protection and, ultimately, her survival.

Here, we see a very young preverbal ego state responsible for the feelings of disgust towards the mother. Since at this age visual images are still missing, they must first be created. This could also be done via artistic means. However, the therapist contacts the ego state "frozen" in defense and disgust, directly on a body level. This "baby ego state" cannot run away from the mother's invasive behavior, and the baby cannot defend herself by kicking, since she depends on the mother for survival. So, there is nothing else for her to do but to remain there, to "freeze," generating tightness and disgust. Both of these are symptoms of the defensive energy mobilized for a flight reaction unable to be acted out and now trapped in the body. This energy can be made to flow and release by attending to it, slowing things down and providing safety. As the therapist stays firm and unwavering, the client and her baby ego state can feel their own power disengaging from the tightness and now feel even more "empowered" through the safe boundaries.

Also, by speaking directly into the system, the therapist informs the baby ego state remaining in the past (Watkins & Watkins, 1997) that the suffering, helplessness, and dependency are over and that it is now free and able to determine by itself what it wants to do. As the baby ego state begins to feel its power, images start arising: The scarab with the golden egg protecting it. The tensed-up baby becomes the golden beetle. This is a clear example of how, by including the body, preverbal ego states can have a lasting corrective experience in a relatively short space of time. In this case excerpt, the baby ego state reaches a higher level of development and with that the ability for imagination.

Subsequently, the physical and emotional effects of the therapeutic sequence are tested with the "body test," that is, the client is invited to remember the triggering situation and to perceive her current body sensations, which are much more immediate than her thoughts. If the client has shifted towards greater relief and relaxation, a step towards healing has been made. Emmerson (2015, p. 61) refers to this as the *imagery check*, when checking the immediately noticeable physical feedback to the visualization of the originally upsetting situation or memory. With the imagery check, you can test whether the situation is now experienced as being emotionally safer, or whether another round is necessary to release all traumatic energy from the system. When, after the treatment, this client mentally re-enters the situation with the symptom, she feels calm and distanced instead of experiencing the intense feelings of disgust.

> . . . *This suggests a clear rationale for a trauma therapy model that separates fear and other strong negative affects from the (normally time-limited) biological immobility response. Separating the two components breaks the feedback loop that rekindles the trauma response. This . . . is the philosopher's stone of informed trauma therapy.*
>
> (Levine, 2010, p. 58)

Change Happens Through the Body

When Ego State therapy is enhanced with body approaches, we can see impressive and lasting changes. Normally, there are clear changes in the inner state towards more settling, reduction of symptoms, and healing, sometimes even quite soon, if the clients are somewhat stable. If we want the effects to last, talking by itself is not enough. The client should *experience* change so that new connections can be consolidated in the brain. First, the "inner feeling" changes, and then the behavior. Current techniques used in Hypno- and Ego State therapy sometimes do not suffice to access immature and undeveloped parts because clients do not have the language or power of imagination. You can see this with Ms. Y. When the body is included, these preverbal states can be accessed directly and easily, and the therapist can communicate with them via the body because body sensations and movements are sometimes the only way for them to express.

Relationship and Safety

The basis for a trusting therapeutic relationship is safety: In order to feel safe, we need a sense of being protected, of control, the feeling that we can have impact and are able to act. The opposite of powerlessness is strength – resilience. And for resilience, self-regulation plays an essential role. The better self-regulation works in early childhood, the healthier and more successful and more resilient we are.

> The pivotal place of self-regulation is made apparent in the results of the Perry Preschool Project, a long-term study over more than 40 years in Michigan, with high risk-children:
>
> The better self-regulation in childhood, the more there is success at school, a higher income, less unemployment, less addictive behavior, less obesity, better health, less criminal behavior in later years (Perkins, 2016).

Even if we as therapists cannot always create the ideal conditions for our clients, or if complete healing is not always possible, we can still help our clients to develop greater balance through better self-regulation.

When the Inner World Seems Dangerous

Clients with a traumatic history, panic attacks, fears, or fatigue depression have difficulties regulating their inner arousal or psychophysiological activation, constantly feeling threatened or under stress. Their organism keeps rating their environment or inner world as being dangerous. Therefore, they try protecting themselves, run away or resist (passively) or they freeze/dissociate.

> A client with experiences of ritual abuse and violence in her childhood and youth by her uncle and aunt cannot deal with the therapist being "too nice." She becomes highly aroused, her body tenses up, she freezes. The "nice" therapist is automatically seen as a danger (a potential perpetrator). At the same time, one or more traumatized child ego states locked in helplessness are activated, overwhelming the client with panic. Immediately, her organism also perceives her inner world as dangerous. The only way out is dissociation. A punishing protecting ego state comes into action. When the therapist speaks to this ego state, it says: "That serves her right. She doesn't deserve better." And: "I hate it when you speak so softly to her!"

This is an extreme example. However, it shows well how dangerous the inner and outer world can appear and how incoherent and insecure the experience of people affected by trauma can be.

The therapeutic relationship creates continuity and *coherence*. By this, we mean that clients can harmonize their body rhythms, such as breathing and heartbeat, as well as their natural body movements or the pulsation between inhalation and exhalation (Schmidt, 2017, p. 168). Through constant coregulation with the therapist, the client can gradually learn to self-regulate and find more stability, both of which are preconditions for the success of a therapy.

Which criteria characterize good therapy? Or how can we measure the success of therapy? Certainly, the subjective way the client feels about life plays an important role. This should clearly differ from when they first entered therapy. But there are also objective criteria:

- Diminution of subjective suffering such as fear and panic attacks, and the somatic symptoms like pain or liability to infections
- Increase in psychological stability, the ability to work, perform and act, and in life energy
- Subsidence of the level of conflicts in relationships
- Return to normal appetite and sleep
- Reduction of addictive tendencies, of aggressive or compulsive behavior
- Brightening of depressive moods towards more life energy and joy
- Stabilization of mood swings
- Reduced urgency and thus frequency of sessions
- More self-respect and self-acceptance
- Coming out of helplessness
- More active coping
- More positive dreams
- Resolving old behavioral patterns.

Playing It Safe: Self-regulation of the Therapist First

Therapists working with traumatized individuals frequently 'pick up' and mirror the postures of their clients and hence their emotions of fear, terror, anger, rage and helplessness. . . if we (the therapists) recoil because we cannot contain and accept them, then we abandon our clients. . . if we are overwhelmed, then we are both lost. If we embody some small portion of a Dalai Lama-like equanimity and 'composure,' we are able to share and help contain our client's terrors in a 'blanket of compassion'.

(Levine, 2010, p. 46)

We already mentioned at the beginning that the therapeutic relationship is one of the most important factors for successful therapy. The relationship starts with the first encounter. Ideally, therapists meet clients in the first interview with an attitude of curiosity and openness, wanting to understand with unconditional positive re-gard (Rogers, 1965).

People seeking out therapy come under psychological strain, worried or even anxious, because they do not know what to expect. They have ventured out of their comfort zone into the unknown and, accordingly, are defenseless. This must be appreciated, just as the fact that every individual is unique must be. Therefore, therapists need to find and create the appropriate procedure for every client, fol-lowing the lead of Carl Rogers or Milton Erickson, by totally tuning into the clients and their concerns, and utilizing the clients' forms of resistance for the therapy (Haley, 2014).

The more safety and trust therapists can already convey in the first session, by meeting the clients exactly where they currently are, listening actively and care-fully, and perceiving clients' body signals and language, the more clients will feel understood and be able to open up to the therapy. At the same time, therapists must track their own body sensations and signals, as well as images, metaphors, and thoughts emerging spontaneously, in order to understand the client. So, on one hand, therapists can be a resonance body ("Oh, so *that's* how the client feels!") and on the other, they can consciously regulate themselves.

Self-reflection and self-regulation are especially important with traumatized, depressive, or strongly suffering clients: If the therapists only "resonate," mir-roring the terror, the pain, and deficits, they fall into the empathy trap. Both therapist and client end up in a *problem trance* (Schmidt, 2017). Peter Levine (1997) would speak about a *trauma vortex*; Steven Porges (1995) of a *fight or flight* or even *freeze mode*. Both dialog partners involved get upset or aggressive and would like to leave the room, or both feel powerless and hopeless, leading to freeze reactions.

Temporarily, compassion and unconditional positive regard cannot be truly au-thentic. If therapists perceive such tendencies in themselves, the art begins: Can they self-regulate in contact with the client by changing their body posture and breathing, on one hand, and, on the other, via abstraction, i.e., a cognitive under-standing of this phenomenon as a countertransference? Can they keep track of clients' pathology and at the same time stay connected to their suffering parts? Therapists protect themselves and their boundaries if they manage to distance themselves, over and over, so they can act thoughtfully from a position of inner observers and persistently "stay on the ball," oriented towards hope and safety (Frederick, 2016).

Of course, this kind of immediate self-reflection cannot always be guaranteed. Still, regular supervision and the knowledge of the underlying psychophysiological processes as described below create the necessary distance. Unconditional positive regard, acceptance, and compassion become possible again.

This is where relationship work happens, with the therapist constantly offer-ing the clients possibilities for a safe coregulating relationship, and teaching them self-regulation through model learning, psychoeducation, and suggesting practical courses of action.

Empathy and Compassion

The psychologist Caroline Falconer, from the University of Nottingham, was able to show that virtual reality therapy can be effective in the treatment of depressive patients. The subjects were equipped with 3D glasses and asked to show compassion for a virtual vis-à-vis. Then they heard their own comforting words. This self-comfort relieved depressive pathology in 9 out of 15 participants (Falconer et al., 2016). Cultivating healthy self-compassion is important even if, in some cultures, it is not always conveyed naturally.

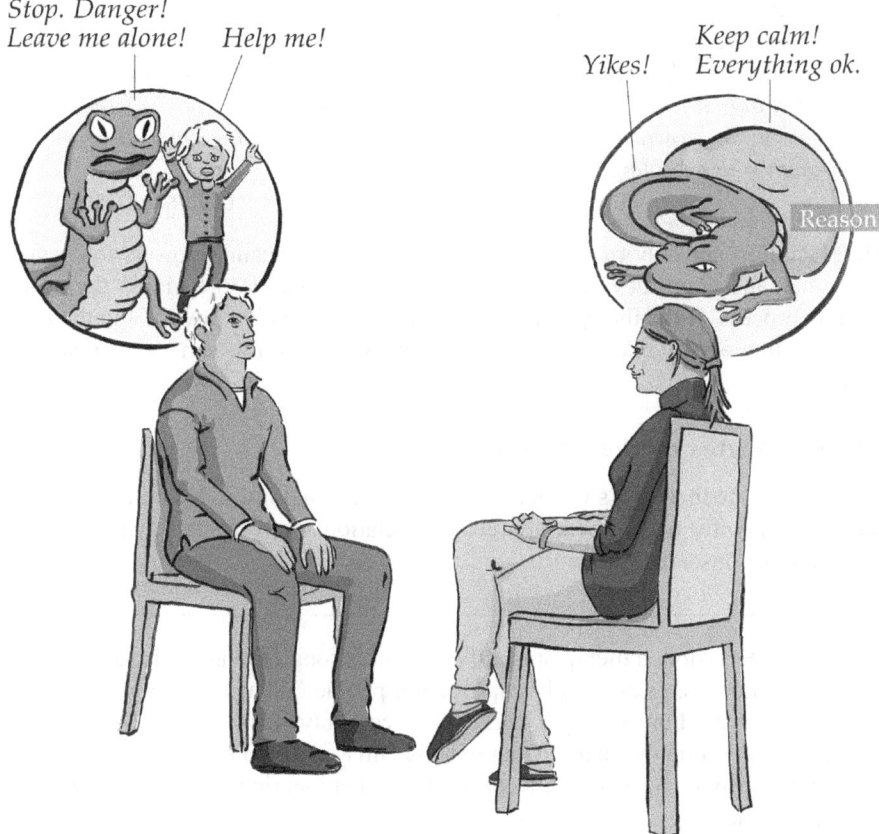

Figure 1.1 Both detect danger. Ambivalence of the client and self-regulation of the therapist in a safe relationship

An "exigent" client, criticizing the therapists and their interventions, is a challenge. Therapists get angry and would prefer to delegate and get rid of the client, a reaction that can be explained physiologically: The therapist's organism automatically and instantly assesses the client's rejection as dangerous and activates defense mechanisms serving self-protection. Here, the personal resources of the therapist come into play. Through self-regulation and self-reflection, the therapist uses their brain holistically so they can gain distance and react paradoxically to the client's hostile attitude. By leaning back to keep track of the whole context, the therapist can show understanding for the client's high demands, while simultaneously passing the ball to the client. The therapist lets the client decide about the next goals, topics of sessions, and each new step in the therapeutic process so that the client always stays in control and takes charge.

Paulsen (2009) refers to a "healing energy field" bigger than the therapeutic alliance:

> *If a therapist feels that s/he must provide the entirety of the energy for the client's healing, there is an increased risk of burnout, as well as a potential for arrogance of self-aggrandizement on the part of the therapist. If the therapist understands an innate healing energy to be an essential part of the human capacity for growth, the therapist's role is reframed as a catalyst or vehicle through which healing may occur.*

(Paulsen, 2009, p. 95)

Here, Paulsen not only refers to incredibly potent self-healing powers inherent in every human being but also to spiritual energy that can be generated during the healing process. If the therapist is aware of these self-healing powers and the enormous healing energy released in a safe treatment context, this can be tremendously relieving.

The Ego States of the Therapist

Sometimes, the therapist's ego states are activated, making it difficult for them to sustain their offer of an open, appreciative relationship, especially when the ego states are unconscious.

After supervision, a therapist is afflicted with strong feelings of inadequacy: "I can't do this. I should give up treating people. What I'm doing is completely wrong. I am wrong!" This deep uncertainty was triggered by the supervisor pointing out that the therapist had missed a step in her intervention, and that also led to strong self-doubts in her therapeutic work with the client she presented.

In the next supervision, the therapist would like to get to the bottom of this uncertainty and agrees to work on it. When the supervisor asks her to imagine being in a position of uncertainty, a little girl appears who has been hurt by her parents' and grandparents' rejection. After having empowered this state, the little one has started to defend herself and do what feels good, the therapist starts laughing cheerfully, her joy spreading: "I am who I am and who I am is good! Just you all look at me!" And she sticks out her tongue. The corrective experience seems to be successful.

After this supervision session, the therapist reports: "I was literally floating out of my supervisor's office. The feeling of not knowing what I'm doing or of doing everything wrong never showed up again. In my next contact with the client (and not only then), I felt totally okay. I am cheerful and sometimes I stick out my tongue! A true moment of glory!"

The Art of Building Relationship

Therapists strive to build a safe relationship and create a therapeutic context that is as pleasant as possible. As mentioned, it is not only important that they try to establish a positive, accepting, and value-free attitude, but also be able to self-regulate and thus protect their own boundaries. This is not only essential for the therapist but also for the client; it is the only way both can feel safe in the relationship. Setting boundaries means that the therapists define for themselves what *they* need to be able to preserve a positive and accepting attitude. It is important to have a therapeutic contract and clear agreements between client and therapist on the conditions of the therapy (what exactly is being offered, keeping appointments, being on time, paying for sessions), as well as clarity regarding the building of relationship. This implies the therapist's persistent presence, which is different from – even the opposite of – merging. A presence with clear boundaries and responsibility for oneself not only provides clients whose boundaries have been violated with safety, but is also necessary for any stable therapeutic relationship. The gift of reliable presence can help to move from defense and dissociation back to human connection. By keeping their own boundaries, therapists are models for the clients. Many people have lost their natural assertiveness, their ability to set boundaries, during their childhood or youth and they must relearn how to do so in therapy.

Knowing about the psychophysiological processes involved, helps both therapists and clients. Therefore, psychoeducation is another important element on the way to self-regulation and integration. It is a great relief for clients to understand that their reactions are normal and are in fact survival strategies of the organism. It helps them to understand and more readily accept themselves. "Oh, and there I was, thinking that something was wrong with me, that I'm bonkers!" is what people often say in this type of situation. Symptoms that were only seen as problems suddenly make sense.

A 16-year-old woman having experienced a lot of violence, neglect, and ruptured relationships in her childhood, is living in a home for children and adolescents. She has to deal with various sanctions because of her aggressive and disrespectful outbursts towards her educators.

In their first meeting, the therapist tries to find out what the client wants to change, but for a start, she is proud of her outbursts because in these moments she feels very strong. Now, the therapist does not try to change her mind but rather to understand what it is like to feel powerful, at least for a short while, accepting and understanding that the young woman does not want to change.

Therapist: I realize you don't want to change those fits, they also give you a sense of strength, don't they? It is more your caregivers at school who want to change that?
Client: (very surprised): Yes.

A little later:

Client: You are the first person who understands me.

In a next therapy session, the client reports recurrent sanctions because she threw another fit, cursing at a teacher.

Therapist: You know what? It might in fact be better for you if you yourself could choose when you want to show strength and when not, no? Then you could decide whether it is worth defending yourself or better to control yourself and put a good face on the situation.
Client: You know, the last psychologist I saw already tried that. It didn't help at all.
Therapist: Oh, I'm so sorry. Let's see if we can find a way.

A little later:

Therapist: It's your birthday soon, isn't it? We could celebrate it in the next session. How would you like to celebrate it? With coffee and cake? What is it you like?

Rather surprised, the client expresses her wishes.

In the next therapy session, the therapist welcomes the client with a small Princess cake (a cream filled cake covered with marzipan) and peach flavored iced tea. The client is pleased, eating and drinking with pleasure. The atmosphere is pleasant and easy. Then, upset, the young woman recounts again about sanctions at school and how she hates being there. She also reports proudly how badly she insulted the educator.

Therapist: If I spat on one half of the cake before you started eating, which half would you have chosen?

The client looks appalled.

Client: Yuck! Certainly the one without the spit!
Therapist: And what would you rather be? A cake that has been spit on or a delicious Princess cake?

The client smiles.

Client: Certainly the delicious one!
Therapist: Exactly. It is so much easier to go through life as a delicious Princess cake; other people simply like you much more. . . . I will now tell you a story; actually, it's a picture book, but I also tell adults this story.

The therapist opens the picture book "Lily, Ben and Omid" (Herzog, 2018) and tells the story of three children and their difficulties. The three of them come to a safe place where a "sweet lady" explains to them why they have these problems. She describes Reason (neocortex), the Antenna (amygdala), and the Lizard (brainstem), and how these parts of the brain function and how their interaction can get out of balance, for instance when the Antenna keeps ringing false alarms, and how some overreact and others always want to remain at the wheel and never give up control. And she shows how the three children can bring their Reason, Antenna, and Saurian back into balance. At first, the client is rather reluctant to listen, but then she gets more and more interested.

Therapist: And now I will show you that this story is not just a fairytale but that Reason, Antenna, and Saurian actually exist in our brain.

The therapist opens the app "3D Brain" (DNA Learning Center) and shows the brain structures in different colors. The client is amazed.

Therapist: You see, it is quite normal that you throw fits so often. Your antenna sounds the alarm and your organism prepares for a fight. Yet we can change these mechanisms in our brain, as in the story, just as we can train different muscles. You can teach your amygdala, your antenna, that it reacts too quickly, like a smoke

> detector already sounding the alarm when a candle has been lit. You can make sure that the saurian does not always remain at the wheel but only in situations where it is really needed. Would you like to try that in the next few sessions?
>
> The client is amazed and agrees.

This example illustrates meeting as equals, meeting the client where she's at, and understanding *her* concern. Moreover, we see how creating a safe context can allow the client to begin to open up to new experiences and developments. It doesn't have to be via a Princess cake or something material. It is enough to meet the clients with appreciative attention, understanding, and interest in them as an individual, interest in their wishes, dreams, needs, strengths, and fears. In the following sessions, building relationship with trust was most important for this client, rather than sophisticated therapeutic techniques. Half-a-year later, it was reported to the therapist that the young woman's manners, behavior, and self-control had markedly improved since the beginning of her therapy.

Orientation and Safety through Psychoeducation

This section points to another requirement for a safe relationship, for successful coregulation, and especially for the stabilization of clients affected by trauma: Psychoeducation. When clients have experienced powerlessness and helplessness, they must understand what happens in their therapy sessions as a part of their therapy. This switches on the neocortex, the precondition for the healing of trauma. For the client, understanding the inner processes creates a sense of control, of normality, and of hope for the improvement of the symptoms. If you consider psychoeducation in the context of an Ego State therapy model, it is to be expected that affected ego states are also listening and can learn.

Psychoeducation must be repeated in the course of the therapy because the client has parts that do not have this information yet or do not have the maturity and ability to understand the information provided by the therapist.

Another aspect in the building of a therapeutic relationship is the creation of a safe therapeutic space, which, however, does not mean that the therapy must always be pleasant for the client or that the therapist can only handle the client with kid gloves. Rather, clients must be encouraged to leave their comfort zone because only then can development take place. Ideally, there is a balance, a movement back and forth between resources and safety on one hand, and the symptom on the other. An intense working phase should not be prolonged, nor should it be intolerable. Clients are invited to venture beyond their comfort zone in small steps. The bigger the window of tolerance, the more confrontation is possible (Sack, 2010).

Anchoring in the Present through Containment

Basically, in trauma, the ability to stay in the here and now is disturbed. Trau-matization means that an experience could not be integrated into one's own past nor represented symbolically. Rather, the experience potentially keeps imposing itself on life in the here and now.

(Ritz, 2017, p. 134)

People possess innate self-healing powers and can, under favorable conditions, self-regulate. According to humanist psychologist Carl Rogers, human beings have an innate drive to grow as individuals and to achieve their full potential. He referred to this desire as the *Actualizing Tendency* (Rogers, 1977). Unresolved posttraumatic stress interferes with these self-regulating abilities, leading to less resilience, the disorganization of the physiology and destabilization, or more suc-cinctly, a very fragile balance.

People affected by trauma and those suffering from excessive fear are haunted by the past and the intrusive feelings, thoughts, and images associated with it, or they are concerned with and afraid of future situations. In therapy, they can learn to increasingly focus on the present. The reader can find many suggestions for how to proceed in Chapter 8 of this book. In order to achieve a higher level of stabili-zation, two factors are essential: Coherence and containment. In this context, *co-herence* implies wholeness, being logical as such, cohesive and comprehensible. In Somatic Experiencing® trauma therapy, a balanced organism self-regulating optimally is called coherent (Levine, 1997). The more coherence clients expe-rience, the more stable they become. Coherence can be determined via breath-ing, heart rate, muscle activity, and change of skin circulation (e.g., from pale to flushed). Using the example of breathing: Hypertonic respiratory muscles limit the natural expansion in inspiration, the breathing becomes shallow and stays above the diaphragm. In contrast, hypotonic muscles do not have enough tone to let natural breathing flow, making for shallow breathing as well. Another indicator of coherence is the heart rate.[1]

A therapist who knows how to self-regulate and is centered, transmits safety, thus facilitating mutual coregulation. However, to reach more coherence, therapists need to be persevering in their accompaniment of the client, part of which is to not only consider common potential, achievable (sub-) goals and looking in the same direction, but also to convey the hope that these goals can be attained in small steps. It is precisely the clients who have experienced attachment ruptures who will chal-lenge this perseverance (cf. the case study in Chapter 3, section on Ego States that Act Destructively).

In Somatic Experiencing®, the term *containment* describes the ability to toler-ate and integrate high energy states by responding to the activation of the sympa-thetic nervous system, and the inner pressure associated with it, with a physical expansion instead of contraction. In this case, the window of tolerance for arousal states increases. Here, the therapist's faculty for containment not only serves as an example (modeling) but is also a necessary precondition. In an unstable organism, without adequate containment, the same coping mechanisms that were involved in the past traumatic situation get triggered, leading to uncontrollable hyperactivation or immobility, freeze, and shutdown.

> The more clients can endure the mobilization of the survival energy trapped in their bodies – i.e., the release of this energy – without being overwhelmed, the bigger their window of tolerance and their ability for containment.

This release of energy can sometimes be quite vehement, which the following case excerpt illustrates.

> The client, Sandrine, has been suffering from chronic back pain ever since she had back surgery seven years ago, limiting her severely and making it nearly impossible for her to sit. She reports having already met the ego state involved in the pain during therapy: A lot has changed and has gotten better, but not nearly enough. She could hardly sit for half-an-hour.
>
> Her current pain level is at 5, with 10 being the maximum, and 0 being pain free.
>
> When the therapist asks Sandrine about her pain and invites her to feel the associated body sensations, Sandrine immediately shifts into a high state of arousal and fear. With a trembling voice she reports about her great fear and palpitation of the heart. At the same time, she reports feeling deep sadness. This reaction comes rather quickly and dramatically.
>
> The currently active ego state is frightened.
>
> *Therapist:* May I speak directly to that part that is so frightened?
> *Client:* Yes.
>
> Therapist What can I call you?
>
> *Client:* Frightened
> *Therapist:* How old are you, Frightened?
> *Client:* Very small, I can't tell.
> *Therapist:* Look at your feet, what do they look like? (cf. Emmerson, 2015)
> *Client:* They are the feet of a baby.
> *Therapist:* Where are you? In a building or outside?
> *Client:* In a corridor.
> *Therapist:* Are you alone?
> *Client:* Yes.

Therapist: Frightened, this is not happening now, it has been over for a long time. Now you are safe. It is a memory in your brain, in your body. It is over. You now have the strength and power to change everything around you so it is good for you . . . I think such a small baby should not be alone, who do you want to be with you?

Client: My parents.

Therapist: Then call your parents. You can have both parents with you, so you are no longer alone.

The arousal increases abruptly, so that the client is breathing rapidly and has a high pulse rate.

Therapist: What is happening now, Frightened?

Client: Papa is not holding me by the hand.

Therapist: Papa, please take your daughter by the hand, she needs you.

Frightened, how is it now?

Client: Mama and Papa are both holding me by the hand.

The client settles somewhat.

Therapist: What do you see?

Client: I see a light at the end of the corridor and a surgery block.

Therapist: I suppose that frightens you and you don't want to go there, do you?

She shakes her head.

Therapist: Like any child, you have the right to be cared for lovingly, to be understood and protected. For some reason, that seems to not have been possible back then. Luckily, it is over now. Now, it is as it should always have been. Now, both your parents are holding you by the hand and are with you. And you deserve that, and always have. It is not your fault that you were so alone. I am so happy that you can now change all that . . . Are your parents still holding you by your hands?

Client: Yes, we are leaving the corridor.

While the therapist is speaking with the client as "Frightened," the client suddenly shows strong physical reactions. She starts shaking uncontrollably, especially her hands.

Therapist: Sandrine, is it okay if I touch you?
Client: Yes.

The therapist takes both the client's hands and holds them, while talking to her both as "Frightened" and to the client.

Therapist: Very good, finally you can let go. I am with you.

She takes Sandrine's feet between her own (containment of hands and feet) and keeps soothing:

Therapist: Breathe, Sandrine. That's it. Very good. Try to exhale very slowly, taking your time. Open your eyes, Sandrine, and look around! Is there something that makes you calm down? Is there something or someone providing safety? (Adult client orienting to the outside, other people, activation of the social engagement system.)
Client: My friend, Susanne. (Susanne is sitting in the training group, watching.)

The therapist asks Susanne to sit next to Sandrine.

Therapist   Please look me in the eyes! (Activation of the social engage-
(to Client):   ment system.)

The client is still breathing fast.

Therapist: Show me with your hand how fast your heart is beating.

The client moves her flat hand over her left breast in the rhythm of her heartbeat.

Therapist: Very good. Now slow down the movement and track what that feels like!

The client slows down the movement, her breathing visibly calming down. Eventually, she stays in a spontaneous hand levitation.

Afterwards, she is immersed in a deep state of trance. The client is a hypnotherapist herself and is very skilled in hypnosis. Later, she reports that she was immersed in a big bright, peaceful light. Her breaths get deeper, longer, and steadier. The therapist gives her time.

Therapist: Please give me a sign when you are ready for the next step.

After a while, the client inhales and exhales deeply and opens her eyes.

Client: Now it's okay.
Therapist: Sandrine, how is Frightened now?
Client: Very well, she is very gentle and sweet.
Therapist: What does Frightened still need?
Client: Somebody explaining to her what's happening!
Therapist: Who could do that? What do I call that part that just said that?
Client: Sandrine.
Therapist: Sandrine, could you explain everything to Frightened and accompany her, take care of her?
Client: Yes.
Therapist: Does the name Frightened actually still fit? No? Frightened, what would you like to be called?
Client: Little Sandrine, I always wanted to be called Little Sandrine.
Therapist: So Frightened has now become Little Sandrine? Isn't that nice? You, Sandrine, and you, Little Sandrine, are not alone, you are now a team. What is the color of your team?
Client: White, the light is so bright.

A gentle reorientation takes place, the therapist giving the client plenty of time.

When the therapist was holding her hands, so the client reports, a great strength and warmth had poured into her. Then, the client had been immersed in that light, being deeply touched by this experience. Her body, having let go everywhere, had no pain anymore but she felt very tired and happy. The therapist asks her to write her an email in a few days to let her know how she is doing. She also makes sure the client does not drive after this intense session.

Half-a-year later, Sandrine reports that, after this intervention, she had felt much better. A month later, she had gone on holiday by plane, spending 17 hours on the plane without any problems, had driven a motor scooter, and gone snorkeling. She was now able to do sports again. There was a considerable difference from what it was like before. She was much more agile and had markedly less pain. And, she says she could often see Little Sandrine holding her parents' hands, smiling at her.

This case excerpt reveals that it is not the content of trauma per se but the client's experience of, and the reaction to, the overwhelming situation that matters. The therapist does not need to know what, for instance, the surgery block is about. Rather, she focusses on bringing little "Frightened" back from the past to the present and helping her to have a new corrective and safe experience. She also focusses on containment, safely accompanying and reassuringly holding and enduring the highly aroused states, as well as on coregulation in the relationship in order to reinforce and increase the client's containment and self-regulation so she can experience coherence. A coherence arising from the integration of "Frightened," who has now become "Little Sandrine," and a part of the inner team, and a coherence on the physical level through the newly developed balance in the organism as well as a corrective relationship experience.

Quite often, as in this instance, intense energies are released when the switch from the freezing mode to the fight-flight mode happens, and, at first, this can be rather unpleasant or even frightening for the clients. (More about this in Chapter 2.) To contain such high states of arousal, a safe therapeutic relationship, containment, and coregulation must have already been established.

With trauma, a coherent experience "falls apart" and remains fragmented. Trauma transformation and integration implies trying to put the fragments of experience back together

(Ritz, 2017, p. 136)

Safety First

Building a safe context needs to happen at the beginning of every psychotherapy, especially with clients who are still unstable, who are suffering from posttraumatic stress, and whose self-regulating capacities are insufficient. By allowing for coregulation on the relational and physical level in the therapeutic contact, clients can increasingly improve their self-regulation, feeling more competent and safer. The central role in healing of safety – and of having a safe relationship to another person – is highlighted in Chapter 2.

Note

1 A healthy, strong heart has a resonant frequency of 0.1 Hz +/− 0.01 Hz. If it beats within this frequency range, the brain can process information more effectively, the immune system functions better. A person who is in a coherent state can influence and calm down other people within a radius of 1.5 to 2.5 meters if they can tune into it.

References

Bion, W. (1970): *Attention and Interpretation*. London: Maresfield.
Emmerson, G. (2015): *Learn Resource Therapy. Clinical Qualification Student Training Manual*. Victoria: Old Golden Point.

Falconer, C. J. *et al.* (2016): Embodying self-compassion within virtual reality and its effects on patients with depression. *British Journal of Psychiatry Open, 2(1)*: 74–80.

Frederick, C. (2016): Beyond Empathy. The Tree of Compassion with Malevolent Ego States. *American Journal of Clinical Hypnosis, 58*: 331–346.

Haley, J. (2014): *Conversations with Milton H. Erickson*, MD. Volume I. *Changing Individuals*. Crown House Publishing.

Herzog, M. (2018): *Lily, Ben and Omid. Three Children Embark on a Journey to Find their "Safe Place"*. Top Support GmbH. https://youtu.be/NozyGLOb5_s?si=5ztwbthWbfd UR6ux

Levine, P. (2010): *In an Unspoken Voice: How the Body Releases Trauma and Restores Goodness*. Berkeley: North Atlantic Books.

Levine, P. (1997): *Waking the Tiger – Healing Trauma*. Berkeley: North Atlantic Books.

Paulsen, S. (2009): *Looking through the Eyes of Trauma and Dissociation. An Illustrated Guide for EMDR Therapists and Clients*. BookSurge Publishing.

Perkins, A. (2016). *The Welfare Trait: How State Benefits Affect Personality*. London: Palgrave Macmillan UK.

Porges, S. W. (1995): Orienting in a Defensive World: Mammalian Modifications of our Evolutionary Heritage. A Polyvagal Theory. *Psychophysiology, 32(4)*: 301–318.

Ritz, P. (2017): Focusing mit traumatisierten PatientInnen in der Personzentrierten Psychotherapie. *Person, 21(3)*.

Rogers, C. R. (1977): *On Becoming a Person. A Therapist's View of Psychotherapy*. Little, Brown & Company.

Rogers, C. R. (1965): *Client-Centered Therapy. Its Current Practice, Implications and Theory*. Gardners Books.

Sack, M. (2010): *Schonende Traumatherapie: Ressourcenorientierte Behandlung von Traumafolgestörungen*. Stuttgart: Schattauer.

Schmidt, G. (2017): *Liebesaffären zwischen Problem und Lösung. Hypnossystemisches Arbeiten in schwierigen Kontexten*. Heidelberg: Carl Auer.

Watkins, J. G., & Watkins H. H. (1997): *Ego states: Theory and therapy*. W.W. Norton & Company.

Chapter 2

Biological Foundations, Theoretical Considerations

Seeking Safety

A sense of safety is vital for our wellbeing and health and affects our whole physiology.

What happens in the nervous system when a person feels safe? According to neuroscientist Stephen Porges (2022, 2009), safety is this physical state that actually enables us to be mentally and socially open, making learning possible. He postulates that resilience arises from the rhythmic alternation between psycho-physiological activation and deactivation by building tension and releasing it in a wavelike motion. Porges showed that this balance can be read from the heart rate variability. The more variable and flexible the heart rate can react in the breathing rhythm, the healthier the organism (Porges, 1995). In the inhale, the sympathetic nervous system comes into play, increasing the pulse, while in the exhale, the heart frequency slows down due to the influence of the parasympathetic. With every breath, the reciprocal cooperation of the sympathetic and the parasympathetic is expressed.

The Social Nervous System

The autonomic nervous system regulates all basic body functions including those of the inner organs. The two branches of the autonomic nervous system, the sympathetic and the parasympathetic, behave contrary to each other and provide the optimal balance between excitation/agitation of the body functions by means of the sympathetic circuit and the soothing/calming/down-regulation of the body functions by means of the parasympathetic. This continuous interaction produces physical and psychological reactions best fitted for the perceived challenges of the environment.

But how does stress change the perception of a person regarding their *social* environment? Neurobiological researchers assume the existence of an *interpersonal neurobiology* (Ogden, Minton, & Pain, 2006). Porges' groundbreaking work described the interaction between the processes in the human nervous system and social behavior in his *Polyvagal Theory* (1995).

DOI: 10.4324/9781003460602-3

Parasympathetic   Sympathetic

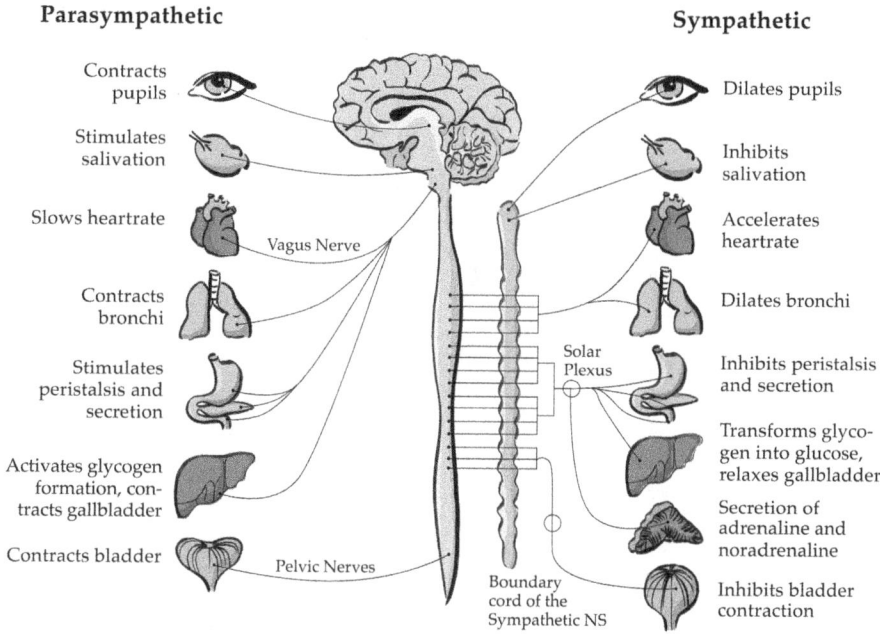

Contracts
pupils   Dilates pupils

Stimulates
salivation   Inhibits
                                                   salivation

Slows heartrate
              Vagus Nerve   Accelerates
                                                   heartrate

Contracts
bronchi   Dilates bronchi

Stimulates   Solar   Inhibits peristalsis
peristalsis and   Plexus   and secretion
secretion

                                                   Transforms glyco-
                                                   gen into glucose,
Activates glycogen   relaxes gallbladder
formation, con-
tracts gallbladder   Secretion of
                                                   adrenaline and
Contracts bladder   noradrenaline
                  Pelvic Nerves
                                    Boundary   Inhibits bladder
                                    cord of the   contraction
                                    Sympathetic NS

Figure 2.1 The two branches of the autonomic nervous system: Sympathetic and
parasympathetic

Porges (1995) postulates that the physiological state has an immediate influence on perception, thinking, feeling, and behavior – and that, inversely, social
events have a strong impact on what happens physically. These processes happen
mainly automatically and involuntarily, below the threshold of consciousness.

The human organism possesses unconscious detectors which can identify
evidence of safety in contact with others, immediately sending signals of self-
soothing to the inner organs. Signals of danger are also identified, entailing cas-
cading physical reactions within milliseconds to activate defense mechanisms.
The process of unconsciously perceiving safety and danger is called *neuroception* (Porges, 2009).

According to Porges (2015a), the key characteristics of social safety are expressed in the interaction of two faces: through a warm facial expression, friendly
eyes, and a pleasant vocal prosody. He believes that connecting to familiar people
is a prerequisite for deep self-soothing, because it requires mutual social interactions and physical closeness (Porges, 2015b).

Here, the vagus nerve, which is part of the parasympathetic nervous system,
plays a crucial role. It is also called the "wandering" nerve because of its branches
all over the organism. It is made up of two branches originating in the brainstem.
Its branches ramify in the area of the head, face, neck, chest, and belly.

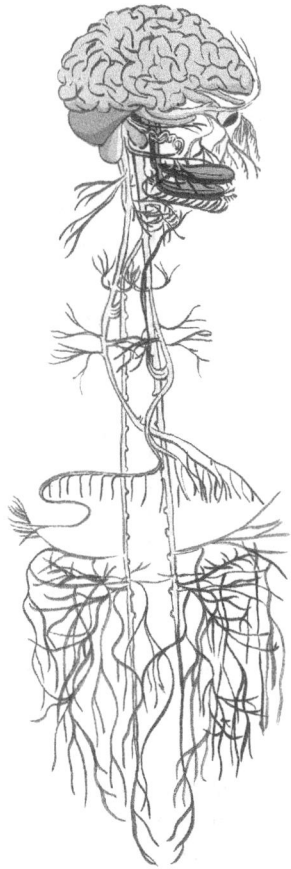

Figure 2.2 The vagus nerve is the X. cranial nerve and the largest nerve of the parasympathetic nervous system. One branch connects to the cranial nerves in the neck, larynx, ears, facial, and mastication muscles, the other innervates the lungs, heart, diaphragm, stomach, and intestines.

The German Nobel prize winner Otto Loewi discovered in 1921 that upon electrical stimulation of the vagus nerve, acetylcholine is discharged, and with that the first and probably most important neurotransmitter, which he named "Vagusstoff."

The Role of Oxytocin in the Social Nervous System

When a person is physically close to people whom the social nervous system, i.e., neuroception, considers to be trustworthy, oxytocin, the hormone associated with trustworthy and safe attachment, is discharged. This happens when closeness is connected with deep muscle relaxation, which Porges calls "immobilization without fear."

The Love Code

The ability to let go in the presence of another person and to relax all the muscles is accompanied by a discharge of oxytocin, but only if the person feels safe and their social nervous system (ventral vagus) is active. This guarantees that muscle tension only releases with physical closeness when the people you are with mean well. The oxytocin acts upon the dorsal vagus in such a way that the person can let go of all defenses and the body can relax deeply. Cradling movements can enhance this effect. Since this quality of togetherness between people allows for attachment, Stephen Porges and his wife, neuroscientist Sue Carter, coined the term the "Neural Love code" (Levine, Porges, & Phillips, 2015).

Oxytocin plays an important role in the social nervous system. Mothers with a high concentration of oxytocin in their blood tend to be especially caring (Gordon et al., 2010). Research shows that oxytocin increases the ability to identify emotions (Lischke et al., 2012). As described, the effect of oxytocin depends on how the context of a situation is interpreted. If very caring parents tend to their children, the discharge of oxytocin in the child is also increased, leading to a safely bonded and emotionally stable child, because oxytocin also has a positive effect on stress regulation in the child's organism.

In principle, the body's own oxytocin reduces stress and negative emotions by increasing empathy and caring attention – especially for members of one's own group (Ijzendoorn & Bakermans-Kranenburg, 2015).

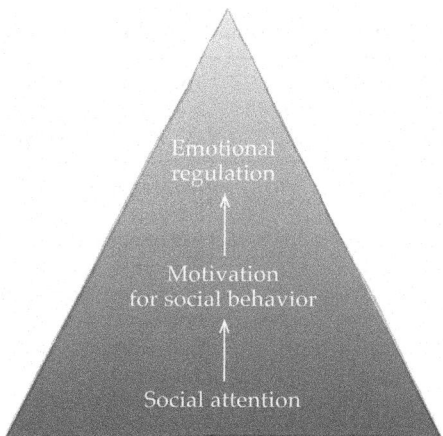

Figure 2.3 The role of oxytocin in the social nervous system

Thanks to the effect of the attachment hormone oxytocin on the reward system, social engagement can be experienced with pleasure, which in turn reinforces the motivation for appropriate behavior. This naturally results in more undivided attention for social interaction given by the salience[1] network. In this context, Strüber (2016) speaks of a model of social adaptation.

The Vagal Paradox

Porges (2009, 2022) investigated the contradictory phenomenon that the vagus nerve not only provides rest but can also have a fatal effect on the organism: The *Vagal Paradox*. He found out that the parasympathetic nervous system is responsible for rest as well as for muscular freeze when we are in great danger. This immobilization that occurs in extreme situations, also known as "fake death," can be associated with respiratory paralysis and lead to death if it lasts too long. When Porges investigated this paradoxical effect of the parasympathetic, he discovered that there are two branches of the vagal nerve with diverging effects on the organism.

The phylogenetically older, *dorsal vagal* part consists of non-myelinated fibers and innervates the smooth muscles of the esophagus, heart, stomach, and intestines. It constitutes a visceromotor component of the vagus nerve.

The younger *ventral* vagus nerve with its myelinated (and therefore fast) fibers not only supplies the visceromotor functions of the heart and bronchi, but also regulates muscle groups related to social behavior, attachment, and maintenance. It innervates the so-called *somatomotor* component; efferent pathways lead to the muscles of the face, masseter, and middle ear as well as to the larynx, pharynx, and sternocleidomastoid. Table 1 shows the different scopes of the two vagus parts.

Table 2.1 Dorsal and ventral vagus complex and their target of innervation

The dorsal vagus complex (pathways unmyelinated) DMNX + NTS (Nucleus tractus solitarii: Nervus VII, IX, X)	The ventral vagus complex (pathways myelinated) Nucleus ambiguous (Nervus IX, X, XI) + Nervus V, VII
Bronchia	Masseter
Heart Muscle	Larynx
Esophagus (lower portion)	Esophagus (upper portion)
Gastrointestinal Tract	Pharynx
	Sternocleidomastoid
	Heart
	Bronchia
	Audition
	Facial muscles

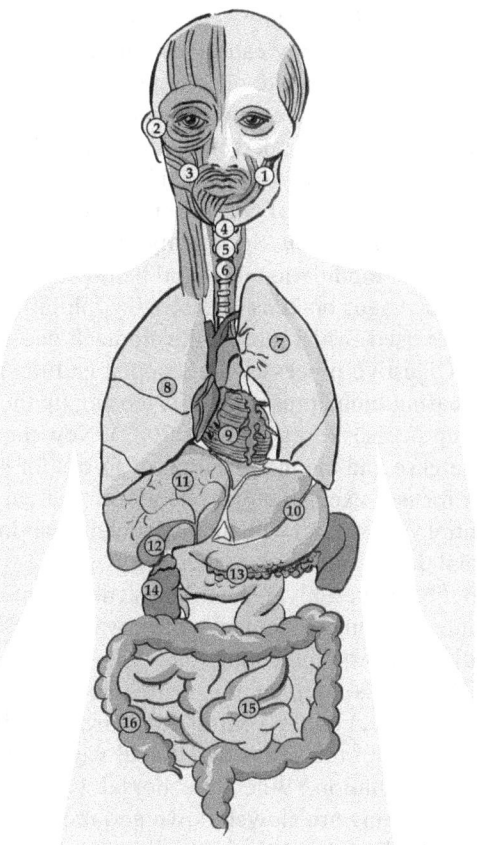

Somatomotor   *visceromotor*

1   Muscles of mastication
2   Middle ear muscles
3   Facial muscles
4   Larynx
5   Pharynx
6   Esophagus
7   Left lung
8   Right lung
9   Heart
10 Stomach
11 Liver
12 Gall bladder
13 Pancreas
14 Ureter
15 Small intestine
16 Upper colon

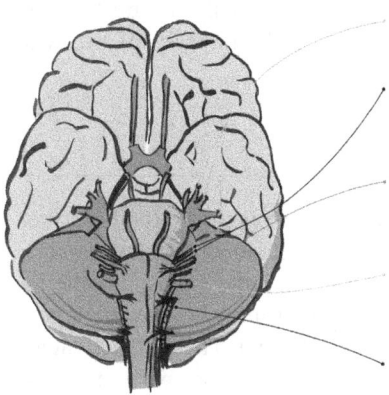

Cranial nerve V: sensory: face, sinuses, teeth; motor: muscles of mastication

Cranial nerve VII: motor: facial muscles; secretory: salivary and lacrimal glands; sensory: tongue, soft palate (taste buds)

Cranial nerve IX: motor: pharyngeal muscles (swallowing); sensory: tongue, pharynx, tonsils, middle ear; secretory: parotid gland

Cranial nerve X: motor and sensory: heart, lungs, larynx, pharynx, palate, trachea, bronchi, gastrointestinal tract; sensory: external ear

Cranial nerve XI: motor: neck and shoulders (sternocleidomastoid).

Figure. 2.4 The ventral vagal complex and its target organs

When the older *dorsal* vagus' tone is in optimal condition there is a pleasant gut feeling and the body can invest energy in food intake and digestion. The vagus nerve acts like a brake on sympathetic arousal. Flight and fight reactions are inhibited, allowing the newer part of the vagus nerve, the *ventral* vagus, to come into effect. Now the person is sociable and emanates a sense of accessibility and playfulness, or shows prosocial behavior, being caring and nourishing, and relaxing in the presence of close friends and family. Porges calls this circuit the *Social Engagement System.* So, the myelinated (fast) *ventral vagal* fibers are responsible for the modulation of social behavior and attachment.

If the vagus brake is released, the inhibition of the sympathetic nervous system is decreased, which upsets the stomach and the gut, leading to fear and/or anxiety. Digestive processes are stopped and the hormone vasopressin is discharged, increasing blood pressure while tensing up the skeletal muscles to initiate flight or fight processes (Porges, 2009, 2022). Now the sympathetic nervous system, aimed at defense and the mobilization of forces for survival, is activated, and the organism focuses exclusively on the ability to fight or take flight. During this time, the ventral vagus – and with that prosocial behavior – is temporarily inhibited, creating social distancing among other things. It goes without saying that this mobilization should only be activated until the acute threat is over, because otherwise the ability to attend to others in a benevolent way suffers, and intimacy and safe attachments could be at risk in the long run.

If self-assertion of the sympathetic nervous system is not successful, the braking effect on the ventral vagus is intensified, activating the phylogenetically oldest part of the vagus, the dorsal vagus. The human organism falls into freeze and dissociation. When the dorsal vagus dominates, the body's metabolism and breathing are slowed down and movements come to a halt, resulting in collapse. In the face of the immediate threat of death, as in the case of an attack by a predator, for example, the dorsal vagus can instantaneously inhibit the activity of the heart and breathing, potentially leading to immobility of the whole organism.

Porges (2009, 2022) summarizes that there are three neural circuits in the mammalian brainstem, having evolved over the course of human history, modulating human reactions: The sympathetic and the parasympathetic nervous system. The parasympathetic is subdivided into the two branches mentioned earlier: The dorsal vagal and the ventral vagal. They are activated in the human system depending on whether safety, danger, or peril to life is perceived. This activation enables adaptive behavior.

Lost in Translation

Via *neuroception*, we not only perceive danger in general but also social signals of threat, such as a shallow, squeezed voice, tension around the eyes, or an aggressive expression around the mouth.

In therapy, you can see that clients who feel subjectively threatened in their social contacts show defensive behavior, making authentic social interactions with them difficult. Such clients tend to automatically distance themselves, showing a flat facial expression, averting their eyes or fixing their gaze, thereby temporarily losing their ability to mirror the facial expression of their vis-à-vis. Emotional resonance is lost and, with that, direct contact is interrupted. Under these circumstances, social contacts become strenuous and unsettling, which in turn prevents the nourishing bonding experiences so badly needed by every human being. If you examine the intra-psychological states of these clients, you notice that underlying defensive behavioral patterns are activated, which are fired by unconscious aversive attachment experiences. Clients in this state will often *overlook* and *miss* important social signals coming from the present in their interactions, making it impossible to introduce corrective experiences that could bring about reassurance. Through such misunderstandings, they miss out on a sense of belonging and security, basic human needs essential for survival. This also happens when possible signals of danger from the environment are overrated or neutral stimuli are misinterpreted.

The Effects of Positive Attention

Fortunately, this is not the end of the story. People who feel this level of threat can learn to open up for social contacts with the help of trainings in self-soothing, specific social interaction exercises, and by learning to distinguish clearly between the past and the present using mindfulness and Ego State therapy. The reactions of the environment, in turn, affect the nervous system of a person. If the vis-à-vis knows how to react in a helpful and well-meaning way, and these signals of safety are absorbed by the individual feeling threatened, the organism calms down and the bonding behavior becomes prevalent again.

According to van der Kolk (2015), a healthy social network of support is the most effective protection against the development of traumatization. Not only sympathy, but gestures such as being held in a soothing way or the feeling of gentle rocking movements communicate to the nervous system that the danger is over. Joint rhythms in dance, singing, or sports and play, and mutual attunement, as described earlier, can all facilitate an experience of connectedness, calming and protecting the whole nervous system. Social games play an important role in this, because they are excellent ways of practicing self-regulation. A good example of this is a mother playing "peekaboo" with her baby: While the mother as the source of safety disappears, the child experiences an arousal of the nervous system, immediately dropping to a pleasant level as soon as the loving face of the mother appears again. In this context, playing can be understood as a neuronal training to practice the neuroception of danger and safety in turn (Porges, 2015b). For these positive effects to be engendered, the social interaction must happen in the presence of the people concerned. Digital games most likely will not have the same effect (Porges, 2015a).

We are Neurobiologically Designed to Seek Attachment

Porges (2017) noticed that the circuit that inhibits defensive behavior is active when there is *connection and harmony with other beings*, a neurobiological correlation of felt safety, allowing for loving human behavior such as compassion, cooperation, and caring. He called it the *Social Engagement System* and defined it as the phylogenetically youngest part of the nervous system, which only develops in mammals and humans. Owing to its efferent fibers, muscle groups that are responsible for social behavior are innervated.

People accessing their abilities for social engagement can be recognized by their facial expression, especially their laughter lines around the eyes and the pleasant prosody of their voice. The social signals they emit invite you to come closer and interact or even play and show that it is not dangerous to get involved with them.

These non-verbal signals happen largely on an autonomous and unconscious level. According to Porges, the muscles involved in the middle ear, face, pharynx, larynx, and neck are innervated by the ventral vagus and are directly connected to the nuclei of the cranial nerves V, VII, IX, X and XI, on the level of the brainstem, as suggested in Figure 2.4 "The ventral vagal complex and its target organs."

Thus, the nerve fibers of the ventral vagal complex influence facial expression, head movements, the pitch of the voice, and listening, and therefore social behavior, the tone of the middle ear muscles filtering human voices out of the din of background sound. When there is a threat, low-pitched sounds are perceived extremely clearly because these are most likely to come from an offender, while high-pitched sounds cannot be filtered out from background noises so easily.

The ventral vagal complex also contributes to affect regulation and inhibit excessive stress reactions, enabling humans and mammals to get attached and approach new situations without fear. Their stimulation leads to whole-body relaxation. This not only stimulates the growth of new brain cells, but also improves memory, sleep, and immune functions, lowering blood pressure and blocking the discharge of cortisol and oxidants. In this way the experience of stress is reduced, and inflammations or allergic reactions are diminished or inhibited.

If the ventral vagus has an optimal tone, i.e., defensive behavior is inhibited, the ground is prepared for *bonding,* the connection between well-meaning people. The activation of the ventral vagus through social interaction, breathing or relaxation techniques, is necessary for the nervous system to settle, and therefore provides the fastest way out of traumatic stressful experiences towards self-regulation. For this, eye contact and turning your face toward the other person are essential, since safety signals are detected by "reading" someone's facial expression. If, through neuro-ception, another person is rated as being safe, the whole nervous system settles.

Overactive Detectors for Danger

As described already, humans and mammals possess a finely tuned sensorium that is constantly scanning the environment for signals of safety or danger. With the help of neuroception, happening unconsciously, the nervous system rates the outer environment and the inner world as being safe or dangerous. Neuroception can neither be deceived by false friendliness nor an artificial facial expression such as a phony smile.

People with complex trauma seem to possess especially finely tuned antenna. They cannot switch off their ability to interpret the quality of voices very precisely. In an experimental study with eight-year-old children, Pollak (Pollak et al., 2000) showed that abused children recognize significantly more often signs of anger or irritation on faces than a control group. Not until neuroception signals safety are defense reactions suppressed. The facial muscles relax, the heartbeat slows down, and (authentic) social contact is possible. Neuroception is often felt directly as our *gut feeling*.

Therapists are well advised to train themselves to notice and define feelings of countertransference as resonance in this neurophysiological process, and then to utilize it accordingly.

The "originator" of this often diffuse gut feeling is, as mentioned earlier, the visceromotor vagus nerve. Zurich researchers (Klarer et al., 2014) discovered in animal experiments that when the afferent fibers to the brain were disrupted during surgery, more recently acquired fears were likely to emerge, but older fear reactions that were already conditioned were more resistant to learning processes. They suspect that innate fear originates from the visceral sensations in the belly area. The authors conclude that a healthy vagal tone is crucial for unlearning conditioned fears.

> *Being able to feel safe with other people is probably the single most important aspect of mental health; safe connections are fundamental to meaningful and satisfying lives.*
>
> Bessel van der Kolk (2015)

When Things get Dangerous: Biologically Inherited Reactions

It is in the nature of humans that tremendous energy is mobilized in the face of danger and challenge, contributing to sparking vibrancy because it expresses our full potential. The brain and nervous system are designed to survive intensive or extreme experiences. Researching flow (Csikszentmihalyi, 2010), positive psychology discovered that feelings of extreme joy, vibrancy, and competence can definitely arise from risky situations requiring top performance. Still, the following aspect is critical: The degree of danger has to be such that the subject feels capable of taking action. This presumption contributes to a sense of competence and has an anxiolytic effect. What happens when the danger exceeds the subjective possibilities? Humans then react like all mammals, searching for help in the environment. Involuntary, biologically innate survival strategies happening autonomously in the human organism can best be observed in gregarious animals in the wild.

Wild animals depend even more than humans on their conspecifics, since there are dangers lurking everywhere. When something unexpected happens, they automatically react with heightened alertness and pause to locate warning noises. With this orienting reaction, they lift their heads abruptly, align their hearing to the source of the noise, and open their sensory channels widely – dominated by astonishment, curiosity, and expectation. If the disruption of the familiar is not experienced as threatening, the animals collect information about their environment with an explorative orienting reaction without being overly activated. However, if the trigger is rated as dangerous, the animals immediately turn to the others to see where they are moving to as they look for the protection of the herd. If the social cry for help by the individual in trouble does not trigger a protective gesture in the group, for instance, because no other animal is nearby, the brain recognizes that it cannot cope with the challenge through the social nervous system by means of ventral vagal activation.

This makes the phylogenetically older survival pattern spring into action, the defensive orienting reaction, where perception is aligned to the sources of danger. If a defense or flight reaction is seen as a worthwhile investment, it is activated through the sympathetic nervous system, entailing a discharge of a high amount of adrenaline and cortisol within a short period of time to create the readiness for a fight. Blood flow to the strained muscles increases and blood pressure rises to provide the muscles with enough oxygen and glucose for the physical effort ahead. Thinking is accelerated and the source of danger located with the utmost alertness. If the animal wins the fight, it experiences triumph and self-efficacy. If fighting is not possible, flight mechanisms are activated. The animal tries to find a way out and uses the energy provided to get away as quickly as possible. If it is successful, body functions normalize and the organism returns to its normal state.

The Biology of Failure

When there is threat to life and fighting seems hopeless and flight impossible, the sympathetic circuit of the autonomic nervous system is inhibited, intense movements coming to a halt. Now, helplessness and despair prevail, and there is freeze to the point of collapse. With the "fake death," the body becomes lifeless and limp, and breathing movements are slowed way down to the point of almost no longer being discernible. This masterstroke of the organism also serves survival: If the prey animal is immobile, the predator tends to turn away from it more easily. The mechanism is due to the strongly heightened dorsal vagal tone of the older branch of the vagus nerve responsible for soothing and regenerating in everyday life. However, relaxation should not be thought of in connection with the freeze reaction, because the parasympathetic, in contrast, is operating full speed. If the survival strategy of freezing is successful and the danger over, the prey animal emerges from the freeze reaction.

Now, all the sympathetic flight energy activated before the collapse is still at its disposal. If, however, the predator does not let its prey go and it is too late for any kind of escape, the prey animal remains immobile.[2] The body's own opiates are discharged, entailing a reduction of pain and numbness of feeling. The psychobiological motor of dissociation is going at top speed as if the soul had to escape the body to remain sound. If death is inevitable, at least pain and fear are relieved with these mechanisms. If this psychobiological immobility lasts too long it can lead to death because of respiratory paralysis.

The Hierarchy of Defense

The three defense systems described are organized hierarchically, the *Social Engagement System* inhibiting the *sympathetic nervous system* via *ventral* vagus in times of peace, and the sympathetic nervous system in turn suppressing the activation of the *dorsal vagal* reflexes. The inhibition also works inversely: If the system lower in the hierarchy is active, the higher circuits are temporarily standing idle. In the case of danger, the lower or phylogenetically older defense mechanisms spring into action and, in a healthy nervous system, are just as quickly inhibited again – once the danger has passed – so that the organism can relax and recover.

Trauma as a Frozen Defense Reaction

In the animal kingdom, the physical reactions of a hunted animal that was able to free itself from the life-threatening situation or to regain consciousness after "fake death" can easily be observed. The highest possible arousal is discharged through involuntary quivering and shaking movements. In his Somatic Experiencing® trauma therapy, Levine (1997) makes the assumption that domesticated animals and humans no longer possess this innate capability to spontaneously discharge high arousal and energy or are prevented from this discharge by their environment or situation. Thus, this is the reason for physical or psychological troubles to occur later, besides the inhibition of the fight or flight actions. For many reasons, the original fight or flight movements are also suppressed in the life of humans.

Therefore, Levine (1997) suggests broadening the definition of trauma and detaching ourselves from the criteria specified by the international classification of psychological disorders that the triggering event causes deep despair in nearly everybody (Dilling, Mombour, & Schmidt, 2000). Instead, he suggests the following definition of trauma: If stimuli from inside or outside (in a small child this can

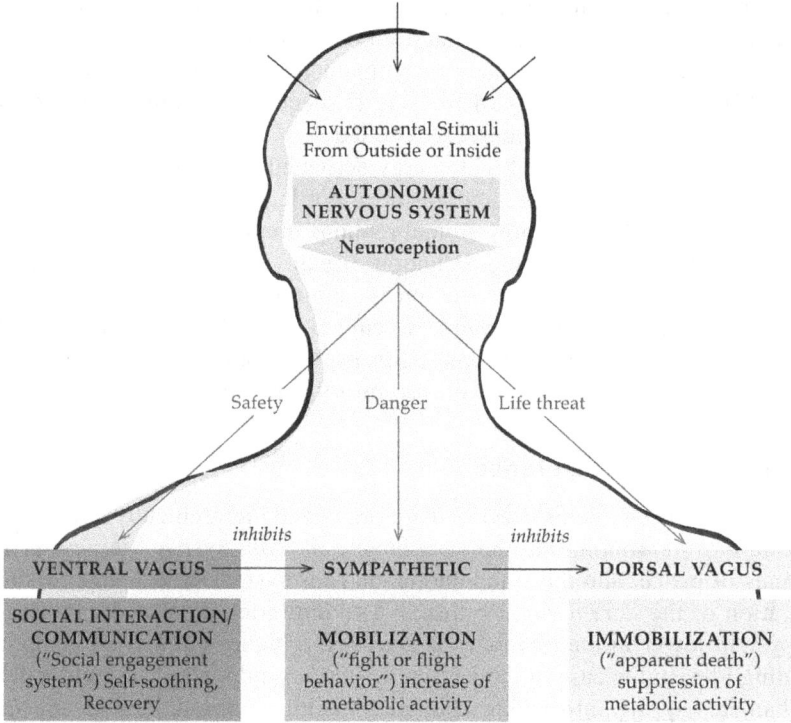

Figure. 2.5 The human defense mechanisms for safety and against threat

be a high fever, for example) act too quickly, too complexly or intensively on the nervous system, overwhelming it, so it cannot react effectively, the organism reacts with helplessness accompanied by physical activation.

As if it were a matter of life and death, all available survival mechanisms and defense strategies are automatically set in motion. It does not even have to be a life-threatening situation. Based on this definition, the *reaction* of the organism to the *perceived* traumatic situation is more essential for the occurrence of posttraumatic stress than the question of whether, objectively, there is a traumatic situation. A shock only results in a posttraumatic disorder if the defense reactions get stuck or cannot be completed, especially the freeze response, but also flight and fight.

For, if the fight or flight actions cannot be completed or the immobility resolved, the energy bound in those reactions remains stored in the muscles, the body freezes or turns numb and cannot be felt. The fairy tale of Sleeping Beauty illustrates this when life (and the whole royal household) suddenly comes to a halt when the princess pricks her finger on a spindle. The water jet stalls and the cook's hand, wanting to box the boy's ears, freezes in midair. This state is anything but passive; rather it is characterized by high muscular activation. Traumatization has occurred if, after the danger has faded, the stress hormones only slowly return to their normal initial level and a state of strong arousal, involving helplessness, continues (van der Kolk, 2015). If it is not possible to take action and to self-regulate within an adequate period of time, the stress reaction becomes chronic, unduly straining the organism in the long run. Sack (2010), therefore, suggests understanding posttraumatic disorders as anxiety disorders.

If a person has been under great stress since childhood, this leads to a neuroception of "constant danger." The environment is experienced as being dangerous and the attempts of others to calm the person are to no avail.

Even if no conscious memory of the trauma is accessible, the body reacts to trigger stimuli related to it as if it were a somatosensory memory with a psychophysiological alarm reaction. With such *implicit memories* (Sack, 2010, pp. 23–27), the same patterns of muscle activation occur as in the initially traumatizing situation. So, it is not the trauma in the past that is the reason for the disorder, but the reactivation of the encapsulated defense reaction brought to a halt back then. Levine (2010) speaks of an *autonomic dysregulation syndrome.*

When somebody reacts habitually to challenges or surprising events with hyperarousal, that is, high arousal and activation of alarm functions of the nervous system, they suffer from flashback-like sensory memories, high sensitivity to light and sound, hyperactivity, nervousness, nightmares, and abrupt mood changes.

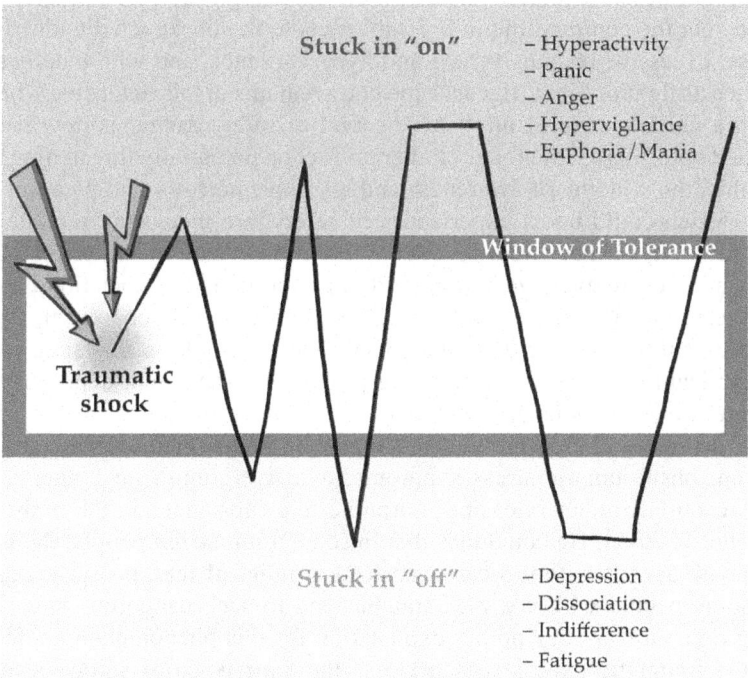

Figure. 2.6 The deregulated nervous system (Levine, 2011)

Stress tolerance is compromised, entailing panic, fear, and psychosomatic stress symptoms. However, with habitual dissociation, such as shutdown or switching off with withdrawal and avoidance, the reaction is trivialization, depression, asthenia, and emotional distancing, leading to chronic helplessness and feelings of lifelessness. Often, the mechanisms alternate, as if a switch was turned from "on" to "off" and back again (Sack, 2010).

False Alarm: The Disadvantages of Neuroception

Psychosomatic troubles can be explained by an imbalance in the autonomic nervous system. When an organism learns to react habitually to stressors with an alarm reaction and flight or fight, a chronic stress reaction with numerous physical aftereffects ensues.

If the sympathetic nervous system dominates, as though the switch were stuck in the "on" position, this excessive arousal presents itself as a tendency to hyperarousal with emotional overactivation, such as fear and panic, anger and hypomania, followed by psychomotor restlessness and tension, having numerous debilitating effects on the musculoskeletal system. The person feels as though permanently having to be on the run or having to defend, the consequence of which are outbursts of anger or moaning, a version of a social cry for help. It is no longer possible to meet unknown or surprising events in a relaxed curious manner. On the contrary, the individual reacts to the unexpected with fright and defense, excessive responsiveness and hypervigilance, and with a defense reaction such as fight or flight. Because the body remains in this defensive worldview, it is in a chronic state of alert. Assessment of safety/danger is now habitually switched onto "high," the focus of attention set on potentially threatening stimuli. With this, the window of awareness and tolerance narrows and pleasant experiences, which could boost experiences of safety, are increasingly made impossible, favoring further stress reactions. Even more fatal is the effect when the organism reacts to aversive stimuli with immobility and dissociation because of past trauma experiences, in other words, with a state of hypoarousal, a psychophysiological collapse or dissociation via freeze. People in this state complain of inexplicable tiredness and digestive problems, exhaustion, depressive states, disinterest, or sensations of numbness.

van der Kolk (2015) pointed out that with some Vietnam veterans suffering from posttraumatic stress syndrome, aversive stimuli no longer triggered stress reactions, rather releasing morphine-like substances in the body, having an analgesic effect. He concludes that in some traumatized people, the confrontation with aversive stimuli can even lead to relief of fear, possibly explaining why some people with complex trauma tend to seek dangerous situations favoring revictimization. Another explanation for this phenomenon could be that repeated traumatic experiences increase the experience of safety because the inner teamwork between ego states is kept up. Both powerful ego states associated with or supportive of the perpetrator and helpless "victim" ego states are validated in their roles and functions through the repetition of the traumatic experience or memory.

As mentioned, unconsciously noticed sensory stimuli coupled with the trauma can also trigger a suitable defense reaction, leading to confusion, fear, or the panic of losing control or even going crazy. People in this condition do not understand what is happening to them, which in turn reinforces the stress and feeling of helplessness. In a life-threatening situation, more memories are stored implicitly through the strong stimulation of the amygdala, so sufferers notice details they would overlook in a normal situation. They experience the events as in slow motion (Eagleman, 2008). Similar to this abundance of details, countless cues in everyday life can re-induce the traumatic memory. For people affected by trauma, it is extremely important that the therapist explains all these mechanisms happening involuntarily. If clients learn that their body and their nervous system actually want to protect them with these symptoms, and that these symptoms are survival strategies that are quite normal as a reaction to shocks, they are gifted with a sense of great relief and reassurance.

Back to the Now: Resolving Traumatic Stress

van der Kolk (2015) arrives at the conclusion that a paradigm shift is happening in modern psychotherapeutic treatment of traumatic disorders because it is not enough to talk about the trauma to achieve resolution of it. Only a few years ago, desensitizing via narrative exposure therapy was considered the treatment of choice in cognitive behavioral therapeutic approaches, whereas today an interdisciplinary approach including many different paradigms is recommended. Herman's work (2003) suggesting differentiating between simple and complex traumatization has raised our awareness that in simple trauma, exposure might be effective, but that with multiple traumatization by close attachment figures, a slower and gentler approach is advisable (Sack, 2010). In the treatment of complex traumatization, holistic therapeutic approaches and international treatment standards should be considered. Further, the cost-benefit-ratio of an affect reactivation first approach should also be weighed seriously in terms of the Hippocratic principle to first and foremost not harm the client (Primum non nocere!), something Martin Sack advocates in his book *Schonende Traumatherapie* (*Gentle Trauma Therapy*) (2010). Today, instead of exploring the trauma in detail, integrative approaches focus on regaining freedom of action and control – the *sensorimotor ability to move and act* – as being *crucial* to free oneself from a dangerous situation (van der Kolk, 2015). In Ego State therapy and the treatment of trauma with Somatic Experiencing®, the focus is also on *the reactions and the experience of the client,* and not on the content of the traumatic experience. Somatic Ego State Therapy stands for a body-oriented approach to obtain an optimal tone of the nervous system, resolve blocked or frozen states and parts, resulting in a full body sense of safety. This cannot normally be achieved with an exclusively cognitive approach.

Creating Physical Safety

Learning requires safety. This means trusting one's own ability to successfully cope with a situation. Only if the organism feels safe, and the ventral vagal path is active via the social engagement system, can the sympathetic nervous system and the dorsal vagus cooperate in a way that health, growth, and healing can be supported and people can recognize themselves as co-creators of their lives. The activation of the ventral vagal system is therefore the only way out of trauma, because it is the circuit in the nervous system not based on defense but on connection. Human nature is designed to overcome precarious situations temporarily, and this takes a stress reaction for the necessary attention and enough energy to be mobilized. In this process, a cascade of hormonal changes is triggered in the brain. If the stress reaction becomes chronic, the hippocampus shrinks, compromising the learning of new information and favoring forgetfulness instead. Imaging methods show that the right prefrontal cortex and the Broca area responsible for language become smaller, which creates deficits in both the working and short-term memory. Similar effects can be found in a posttraumatic stress syndrome, depression, and chronic pain. Fortunately, these effects on the hippocampus are reversible when the stress is suspended. Mindfulness-based relaxation procedures and gentle body work, applied regularly, are therefore effective methods to bring the nervous system into balance and create a protective shield against chronic stress or pain (Emerson & Hopper, 2014). According to Levine (2015), it is particularly helpful to calm the organs below the diaphragm, e.g., with Pranayama yoga or mindfulness meditation, where the emphasis is on *slowing down* exhalation.[3]

For people with posttraumatic stress symptoms, timely therapeutic treatment is indicated, because as long as freezing or dissociative states paralyze the organism, access to resources is impeded, so that growth processes can be delayed or missing. In immobility, the organism releases opiates and endorphins in the face of a threat to protect itself from pain. Hence the dissociative state can be very pleasant for people concerned, yet it comes at a high cost. The more often such phenomena occur, the more unstable, insecure, and helpless people become. Vitality and expansion are barely possible over time.

The immobility reaction occurs when the defensive reaction, such as fight or flight gestures, was not successful or was prevented. If this physically manifested freezing is resolved with body psychotherapeutic methods, e.g., with Levine's Somatic Experiencing® method (1997), the frozen defensive reactions are diluted and brought back to life. Now, all of sudden, intense physical energies are available that were bound before in the state of immobility. As in the case studies mentioned in the first chapters, clients report feelings of "strength" and a sense of "empowerment."

A traumatic discharge . . . converts blocked trauma energy into vitality, into available life energy. Seen in this way, we are not talking about "healing" the trauma, but about "transforming" the trauma into vitality.

(Ritz, 2017, p. 137, translation by S. Zanotta)

The therapeutic process centers less on narrative content and more on freeing the organism in a straightforward way from its straining overcharge and helplessness, by slowing down motoric defense actions and completing them in the presence of the therapist. The focus is on slowing down and pausing, as well as imagining movements, not acting out. If this controlled, carefully dosed transformation is successful, the person experiences an immediate relief, feeling alive and able to act. Experience shows that with accurate preparation and attention to timing a clear change in the client's state can be realized in just a few sessions.

I feel much more whole. Only now do I notice how one-sided I was. Now I am present with both sides. Sitting is much more pleasant. It feels as though my inner parts have returned to my body.

(51-year-old female client)

However, this procedure should not be equated with the kind of emotional abreaction accompanying the release of painful emotions after a mere reactivation of a traumatic memory, as is applied successfully with simple traumata.[4] In modern therapies, inducing an abreaction is no longer the primary objective of the therapeutic work. Somatic Experiencing® trauma therapy simply modifies the reaction to the trauma (Phillips, 2014).

Transformation: From Immobility to Vitality

Somatic Experiencing® trauma therapy according to Levine (1997) is well suited for a slow and gradual approach to resolving a state of freeze. It can be used in all stages of therapy to complement Ego State therapy and is capable of reaching far into the deeper and more unconscious processes of the nervous system, where words alone cannot. With kinesthetic, sensory-motor or sensory processes, neuronal homeostasis can re-settle. Here, changes happen by the non-verbal experience of inner body sensations (interoception) and the conscious orientation in space (proprioception).

When coming out of a freeze reaction, an acute onset of high activation is to be expected, as described in the case study with little "Frightened" in Chapter 1, because only now can the fight or flight impulses that were frozen in the initial sensitizing situation be released (Levine, 2015). The therapist makes sure to clear the way carefully and mindfully, so that these forces can be expressed cautiously and in small doses with physical micromovements in slow motion, thus releasing the tension. This process is called *titration* (Levine, 2015). That way, overwhelming sensations and feelings are divided into small pieces so that the body can "digest" and integrate them. It is important to pause and stop so clients can notice their body sensations and name them: "*How/what is it like now? What is happening with you?*" Since most clients are not used to naming body sensations and therefore it is difficult for them, the therapist supports this process (see instructions in Chapter 8, "Learning to Name Sensations") by suggesting contrary sensations like in a multiple-choice procedure or multiple selection, which the clients can usually answer quickly. This can help clients find words for what they feel.

The Remedy of Bonding and Connection

Based on what was described in the last section, one might think that traumatic experiences only resolve on the physical level, but this is not the case. Trust in the therapeutic alliance is key for this process. Without a person of trust able to hold, accompany, and limit the high sympathetic activation, there is no coregulation – and thus no self-regulation can happen. A firmly established practice of self-care is therefore essential for any therapeutic expert. How the therapist witnessing traumatic events over and over finds a harmonizing balance for body and mind in their time off is, of course, an individual choice. Some find balance through exercise such as yoga, Tai Chi, karate, dancing, or hiking; others prefer meditation, mindfulness exercises, music, connecting to nature or animals, or spirituality, etc. Mindful self-care and self-regulation competency enables trauma therapists to maintain the grounding function of containment, even when the client is in a state of high arousal (Levine, 2015).

A state of high physical arousal can settle via the social engagement system – mainly eye contact, a calming voice, accurate accompaniment of movements, or walking around in the room, sometimes even through specifically applied touch. One of the unpleasant consequences of trauma, freezing, and powerlessness, is this feeling of losing connection – to oneself, to one's body, and to the environment. One feels alien, cut off from the world, out of place, withdrawing, and falling into isolation. Children are especially prone to cutting themselves off, because they have fewer social resources and have not yet fully developed their defense and coping strategies. If, in addition, there is a distorted social perception, the interactions between people and also between ego states can no longer flow without hindrance.

Thus, clients should be supported in reestablishing the connection to the body but also to the environment, to goals and resources – and to other human beings. Social support is the dominating factor for the prevention of posttraumatic stress syndrome. Safety signals coming from other people support coregulation (Phillips, 2016). Part of this is also an objective shared by client and therapist. It is only possible to draw and preserve hope if both are looking in the same direction (for a solution) and if clients can physically feel hope. This is facilitated by jointly defining the objective and examining the therapeutic path from start to finish. The client can stand there and experience what it will feel like once the end has been reached. The possible change can be felt and experienced physically (Beaulieu, 2016).

Touch in Psychotherapy

In psychotherapy, touch is off-limits; in some countries it's even prohibited by law. These rules serve as a protection for the client. Still, in specific situations, touch can be healing, but only with clients who feel safe in the relationship to the therapist, who have not suffered from a violation of their physical boundaries in the past, and who agree.

The question of "touch" must be clarified with clients, and before any touching intervention occurs their permission must be sought. It is imperative for therapists that they know exactly what they are doing; that is, what the precise effect of their touch is. This is why, in my opinion, touch in psychotherapy is a delicate matter if you do not have suitable body psycho-therapeutic training, e.g., Somatic Experiencing® trauma therapy or Somatic Ego State Therapy. If clients are overwhelmed by intense feelings, such as grief or fear, touching at the upper arm or the shoulder can be healing, since this immediately reestablishes the ventral vagal connection, which is especially helpful in early trauma, because it can provide a corrective experience, signaling: I am with you, I'm staying in touch. Humans are social beings, withering without social contact. The therapist can ask the client: "Is it okay if I touch you here at your upper arm or your shoulder?" The case study in Chapter 1 shows how important timing and continuity are for this big shift.

Continuity, in this context, means that with a connection between present and past, there is a thread with which the information can be reorganized and decisions can be made (Levine, 2015). The 52-year-old female client in the case study in Chapter 1 describes how stabilizing and healing touch at the right moment can be:

Through the touch on my shoulder, I came back into my body, and that was an Aha! moment: 'Oh, yes, I am here!'

Therapists without appropriate training can invite clients to touch themselves and explore the resulting body sensations: "Would you like to try out what it is like to put your hand on this part of your body? What does it feel like? Maybe it would be more pleasant to touch yourself somewhere else?" Or the therapist can make specific suggestions: "Put one hand on your sternum, the other on your belly, above the navel. How is that? Take time to feel into it and notice, what it is like now?" "Hold both upper arms, squeeze a little bit, what's that like?" Another possibility is to use a cushion or shawls for support or boundaries.

Social (Re-)Learning in Therapy

As we have seen, psychotherapy ideally induces holistic learning. In multimodal Hypno-somatic Ego State therapy, renegotiation of the client's history not only happens on the physical level, but also psychologically through corrective experiences, both *within* the therapeutic relationship and *on the inner stage* with the client's relevant ego states. Via coregulation and psychoeducation, clients learn at the beginning of the therapy to self-regulate and thus connect to others again. The social interaction in psychotherapy is a quasineuronal training of the social engagement system and a requirement for the healing of trauma.

Ego states can be active in all three systems – the sympathetic nervous system, the ventral, and the dorsal vagus. The dorsal vagal freezing reaction is a great challenge in trauma therapy. It can be resolved by focusing on, and activating, movement and action. Therapists support and accompany, carefully tracking motor impulses for movement and action and ensure that the client comes out of the passive freeze into activity. At the same time, they help the ego states involved to have corrective experiences by identifying their strength through defense and finding their way from the past into the present. Particularly at the beginning of the therapy, the focus is on being present and supporting the client's basic life functions and self-care in everyday life; that is, their attentiveness to physical sensations and needs is primed and their ability to act is strengthened.

Regulating Comes Before Exploring

Psychotherapy should not happen exclusively at the verbal or cognitive level. It is even advisable to work more on the body at the beginning of the therapy with the objective to promote self-regulation. If trauma is explored with detailed questions too early, immediate defense reactions might be triggered. Before deepening biographical content, it is helpful to support the client's body in being able to complete sensory processes and coming into the present. Clients need support in grounding their awareness firmly in the present and experiencing themselves therein. Phillips (2016) points out that traumatized people are afraid of their inner world and, therefore, of exploring their feelings or even their body sensations. For clients with complex trauma, it is crucial to build trust in the relationship to the therapist at the beginning of a therapy, so they can feel safe in the therapeutic space. The therapist shows the clients how to self-regulate, which paves the way for them to steadily improve their self-regulation through coregulation. In doing so, clients should be encouraged *to stay in their experience of the present* rather than in the past. The therapist must recognize signs of deregulation, too much activation, or states of arousal early and interrupt these processes before they overwhelm and compromise the client. Once trust has been established, the therapist may start to pique the client's curiosity around inner experiences, to explore fears in this regard and to carefully challenge them. This can be a lengthy process, during which only small steps are possible. Clients keep the control and the responsibility for the pace and rhythm of the therapy, while the therapist encourages them to leave their comfort zone temporarily and try something new.

For stable people, cohesion and continuity are a given. Cohesion describes the level of coherence of psychological experience, the integration of behavior, feeling, sensory experience, and cognition. This quality relates to the integration of an experience. Cohesion is the opposite of fragmentation. Continuity (Levine, 2015) relates to chronological coherence, the thread connecting the past with the future: We will be more or less the same tomorrow and will still be here. For clients with a dissociative identity disorder, the continuity of daily routine is not a given. Time and again, there can be dissociative experiences with memory gaps. In therapy, the focus is on promoting continuity and cohesion.

A client with a dissociative identity disorder reports in his weekly sessions exactly and chronologically what he has experienced in the days between the sessions. The therapist accompanies the accounts carefully and mindfully, pointing to developmental steps and resources and guiding the client with questions to help him pause and to explore present experiences. "What is that like for you now, when you tell me that?" In this way, the client can develop more continuity and coherence, he is given more control over his life as a chronological experience, and with that more stability.

Moreover, with Ego State therapy, we have the possibility to form alliances on the inner stage, connecting weak ego states with strong ones, or to strengthen the whole personality with concepts of the *indestructible core self*, "inner strength," "inner wisdom," "inner healer," or the "conflict-free self." Also, accessing ego states with the "Dissociative Table Technique," originally suggested by Fraser, or the "Conference Room" (Paulsen, 2009) can be done early in therapy to strengthen resources. To start with, helping, supportive personality parts are visualized for stabilization and invited to the round table. The client's ability to dissociate is utilized hypnotherapeutically. This can also be done by using the "inner observer" or taking a bird's eye view.

A 30-year-old client, familiar with some of her ego states, is suffering from regularly occurring stomachaches. The therapist asks her to describe them. The client has a hard time naming her body sensations and so the therapist asks for a figure, an image, or a word that would fit. The client compares her stomachache to a black volcano. When asked by the therapist what might help, the client can't find an answer. The therapist offers, "Maybe one of your resources knows more? Who could help?" But they also do not know, whereupon the therapist invites the client to imagine leaving her body and looking at the volcanic crater from above, taking the position of an observer or a bird's eye perspective. "What does it look like from up there? Are you far enough?" From the observer's perspective, the volcanic crater undergoes a change.

Client: The crater must be filled with water.
Therapist: Wonderful. Take your time, until the crater is filled with water . . . what is it like now?
Client: It's nice. All my strong parts are reflected in the water and are forming a star. That is good for me.
Therapist: (giving her time) What's it like now?

Client:	The hole is gone. I still feel a little pain in my body.
Therapist:	What else can be done for your body? – Take your time. Your organism knows what it needs, you just have to give it time.
Client:	(after a while) There is an underground source flushing out the pain.

Besides bringing a sense of achievement, this intervention also enlarges the client's window of tolerance. In other words, the client can tolerate high states of arousal more easily, so that therapist and client can address the exploration of more difficult issues and inner life, enabling new liberating inner experiences.

In this process, the focus is not on the content of the narrative, but rather the concrete experiences involved. Psychoeducation is another helpful element for people affected by trauma.

Knowing What is Happening to You

Clients suffering from defensive patterns ambushing them automatically in inappropriate situations, are relieved to know that this is not about randomly controlled physiological processes, but that the brain functions just the same as it did two million years ago: When there is a threat, involuntary mechanisms happen, the amygdala raises the alarm, the body switches to fight or flight. If it is prevented from doing so, it freezes. This occurs before conscious thought taking shape through the neocortex can explain what is happening, collateral damages included. The provoking triggers are most often unknown. Well-meant gestures of the therapist can spark petrifying fear and anger.

If the neurobiological processes are clearly explained in the context of psychoeducation, the potential for self-deprecation is decreased and the space for hopeful expectation is increased. It is a great relief for clients to hear that all humans possess these mechanisms and that they are normal, absolutely necessary survival strategies of our organism. It is worth pointing out that it is possible to use psychotherapy to contribute indirectly to reducing such overreactions.

Once clients realize on a cognitive level what has happened to them and that their organisms only wanted to protect them from a (perceived) threat to life, they will likely experience relief.

Experiencing First, Talking Afterwards

In order to learn to self-soothe, psychoeducation is needed, but before that an understanding of inner processes through experience lays the groundwork. For the client to *grasp* how the body is reacting – and to what – on a sensory level in the here and now, Somatic Experiencing® works with integral inner sensations and resources in the present. Here, the so-called *felt sense*, a term coined by Eugene Gendlin in the context of Focusing therapy (Gendlin, 2003), plays an important role. In Focusing, one's attention is focused on the body, trying to stay in contact with all parts of one's experience and perceiving benevolently what is happening and what one feels or suspects to be meaningful. This results in thinking and healing steps. Focusing can also mean turning one's attention to the physical discomfort associated with a problem. The thinking steps leading to insights and solutions are activated and accompanied by the felt sense, a holistic experience that is new and unexpected. An example of this is the "gut feeling" in a bad situation without knowing what the exact meaning is. The felt sense can only be felt when given the opportunity to unfold with complete mindfulness, presence, and unintentionality in the present moment. The felt sense is also central in Somatic Experiencing® trauma therapy, because physical sensations are explored as well, leading spontaneously to expansion, recognizing resources, and problem solving. Visual notions and the course of movements are explored, with cognitive and emotional processes being given less importance, though they do have a certain significance. The Somatic Experiencing® approach helps in re-regulating the autonomic nervous system by restoring the gentle cycles of the interplay between the sympathetic and parasympathetic and thus boosting the self-healing powers of the organism. Working with a careful dosage, "just enough" activation is used to enable a discharge, an integration and/or a completion within the client's momentary scope of resilience, When a person's tolerance towards their physical sensations gets bigger, they learn to trust the inner wisdom of their body and start uncoupling *in the present* the fear and terror they experienced during the event *back then*, thus gaining emotional distance from the aversive experience, with psychic self-defense mechanisms such as dissociation no longer being necessary. The corrective experience also happens on the somatic level.

From Violation to Rewiring and Connection

As a help for the therapist, Levine constructed what he calls the SIBAM model (Levine 1991), a model serving orientation and intervention on a meta level, to better support the client in connecting or differentiating experiential elements, if necessary, to soften the impact of activation and complete integration of the traumatic experience as a whole.

The model helps to discern which channel of human experience the client is actually moving on and whether all dimensions of experience were involved in the therapeutic process: From **S**ensations, **I**magination to **B**ehavior, the focus of attention wanders to the **A**ffects and **M**eaning. On which channel can clients be reached? Where do they experience their greatest challenges? How can the different elements of experience be related to each other? Regardless of whether you proceed more strategically or intuitively, with this model one can check periodically whether all elements of experience have been considered and where an unerring intervention can be made to facilitate a vital difference in the experience of the client. This kind of procedure accompanies clients through the whole range of their experiences, fostering rewiring and connection between different areas of the brain and facilitating the re-storage of stressful memories.

Clients discover themselves by exploring feeling and movement, thoughts and convictions, all three parts of the brain being addressed, as well as all three parts of the nervous system.

The "Triune" Brain Model[5]

At the core of human identity are sensory sensations coming from the depth of the viscera, the enteric nervous system. We can also speak of the gut's *second brain*. People noticing those sensations deep within the body feel the aliveness of them. "I feel, therefore I am" (Damasio, 2021). Eighty percent of the exchange of information between gut and brain runs bottom-up and is transported from the abdominal viscera through the vagus nerve into the brainstem. Top-down processes from the brain into the gut only make up 20 percent of the information. The language of the reptilian brain is sensations. If you want to communicate with it, this is only possible through actions modulating the visceral sensations! Thus, clients can learn to perceive their sensations and to interact with them skillfully.

The *reptilian brain*, as the oldest entity, controls all processes concerning the immediate survival of the organism and its reproduction. Moreover, it regulates the basic physical reactions to stress or threat, hence the motoric execution of the fight or flight reflex as well as the freeze reaction. When watching reptiles, one notices that they behave in an energy-saving way. Apart from food intake, they hardly move and their breathing is decelerated. Humans also possess this energy-saving program from primeval times, springing into action with the dorsal collapse, i.e., the immobility reaction described. The reptilian brain is steered by reflexes that are resistant to change, being solidly programmed into the hardware of our system.

The second and phylogenetically younger brain is also called *mammal brain*. Here, the midbrain with its limbic system regulates bonding and brood care behavior through emotional processes such as anger, sadness, joy, and feelings of happiness (cardiovascular system). Via this brain, a felt connection to conspecifics is created (belonging, connection, attachment). "I love, therefore I am." Because it is connected to the memory through the hippocampus, basal social behavior patterns can be learned here.

Traumatic stress repeatedly triggers defense reactions through the amygdala, the alarm control center of the limbic system. With sensory information, which is being compared to familiar experiences from the past in the thalamus, the reaction of the amygdala tints the emotional meaning of an event. The hippocampus decides whether and where this experience is stored, so experiences are organized not by content but by affect. Therefore, the reactions and *experiences* of the clients are essential for therapy, not the content of a trauma.

The *neocortex*, our head-brain, with its frontal brain functions, permits higher functions such as abstract thinking, cognition, problem solving, planning, and strategic reaction to new challenges. "I think, therefore I am," is the first proposition of philosopher Descartes. The cognitive functions allow for thinking, abstraction, reason, analysis, and meaning through language, metaphors, and symbols. With the help of the neocortex, humans can tell a coherent story and control their perception consciously.

When all three brains cooperate and the neocortex is actively involved, reintegration of experience (i.e., learning) can happen through the conscious mindfulness to inner sensations. Psychotherapy should allow for that, if it wants to work in a brain-compatible way. Above all, it is essential to support clients in training their executive role outside of therapy to improve their self-regulation and self-management. With the Somatic Experiencing® method, all parts of the brain and all three parts of the autonomic nervous system (dorsal vagal, sympathetic, and ventral vagal) are included and involved. The optimal functioning of the autonomic nervous system is restored

Table 2.2 Following the heart, trusting the gut feeling and keeping track with the mind

Head, Heart, and Gut Brain in a Nutshell
Neuroscientists discovered complex neuronal networks in the human cardio- and entero-systems, which can be described as "brains" regarding their function. In the gut, there are more nerve cells than in the spinal cord, and the same neurotransmitters are discharged as in the brain. As of late, it is known that the heart functions are also regulated indirectly through nerve cells in the anterior hypothalamus, involving thyroid hormones, as shown by Jens Mittag and his research group (Mittag et al., 2013).
Primary Functions of the "Gut Brain"
Here, core identity is provided through sensory perception: "I am." The core self is *experienced* via visceral sensations. The gut brain serves self-assertion, self-protection, and setting boundaries. It helps people recognize their likes and dislikes. This is where mobilization, movement, and activity originate. It is the seat of courage and willpower.
Primary Functions of the "Heart Brain"
Emotions such as anger, sadness, joy, and feelings of happiness, etc., orient toward one's own dreams and wishes and reveal the values one holds: "I love." Emotions relate to the connection with others, expressed with love, hatred, indifference, compassion, disinterest. Via the condensate of these feelings, the degree of sympathy or antipathy for another human can be assessed.
Primary Functions of the "Head Brain"
All processes related to reason, perception, cognition, and regulation, happen in cooperation with the head brain. Thinking, cognition, abstraction, analysis, and meta-cognition help in giving a meaning – semantic processes, language, metaphors, symbols, and higher cognitive activities: "I think" (Phillips, 2016).

by non-verbally experiencing inner body sensations, whereby three strands of body perception are being interwoven: The sensory experience that is directed inwardly (interoception), the sensation of orienting in space (proprioception), and the experience of movement (kinesthesia). Not before these three experiential resources have been experienced in the body by being perceived, and the autonomic balance strengthened through self-regulation, can trauma-related fight or flight reactions bound in the body be activated accurately. Relevant reaction chains are dissolved in small steps, by decelerating them into micro movements and interrupting them by pausing and noticing what occurs repeatedly, so they can be acted out in a controlled and safe way.

Table 2.2 illustrates that psychotherapeutic interventions are based on a holistic approach and should involve the whole brain as much as possible in order to facilitate learning processes. According to van der Kolk (2015), creating relationship through social support is the most important criterion for trauma healing. With self-regulation and coregulation the ground is prepared for the resolution of fight, flight, and freeze reactions with Somatic Experiencing® techniques.

The therapist accompanies and supports these processes mindfully, reassuring clients when severe body reactions frighten them. This corrective experience on a physical level is constantly being combined and complemented by interventions used in Ego State therapy. The therapist can activate or suggest protective allies, if there are any that are already known, bring emerging injured parts into the present, strengthening and integrating them, and bring in destructive states and use them as supportive energies so that, due to these corrective experiences, wholeness can also be attained on a psychological level. Phillips and Frederick (1995) speak of the healing of the divided self.

A 40-year-old female client, with many years of psychotherapeutic experience, still feels strained by her traumatic childhood involving loss and parentification. Younger problem-related parts are brought into the present right from the very first session, using interventions from Ego State therapy, and then they are strengthened, relieved, retroactively nourished and integrated. Moreover, clarifying conversations with important family members are held on the inner stage, and these are also nourished retroactively.

After the first session, the client already reports: "That was a very impressive session, where freedom and space developed inside." In the fourth session, an 11-year-old ego state is retrieved from a situation in which a grandfather overstepped boundaries and led to a cozy bungalow with carpets and banana trees, with a kitten, parrots, a dog, a nice woman, an ideal Mum ("surrogate mum") and an ideal brother.

Her feedback at the beginning of the fifth session: "It's amazing how much has settled in a short time, with a lasting effect on a deeper level."

This is also expressed in outside reality. The symptom, inexplicable anger at her partner, is gone. The client no longer feels powerless, and she has more energy for other things.

However, the client also notes that she keeps experiencing massive setbacks in her self-worth. When nurturing another younger part involved, headache and nausea develop and do not disappear after the intervention. The therapist asks the client to stay with these unpleasant sensations for a moment: "What do you notice?" "I feel dirty, debased, not okay!" These feelings are related to a nine-year-old ego state called Vera. Vera had appeared earlier and had been "saved." For the therapist, either Vera's suffering had not been acknowledged enough or she does not feel quite safe yet. She asks the client whether she could speak to Vera directly. Having obtained her agreement, she says: "I'm now talking to you, Vera. I've heard that you feel dirty, not okay?" The client nods.

"Is there something you have not told your grandfather yet? That he should leave you alone, that your space belongs to you?" She nods. "Tell him directly!" Whereupon the client as Vera says: "Leave me alone, I want you to go further away. You're coming too close to me. You're an asshole!" The therapist supports her: "Very good. Just speak out and tell him what you think! At last you can do it! You are precious and have the right to defend yourself!" After Vera has told her grandfather everything that is on her mind, the therapist asks: "Now, would you like to keep Grandfather in your inner space or would you like him out?" Vera no longer wants the grandfather in her space and sends him out of her inner space, with loud exhalation and hand movements and the support of the therapist. Accompanied by the adult client, little Vera visits a waterfall, where she clears herself from dirt and disgust. Then Vera receives a fur coat as a "safe boundary," protecting and strengthening her.

At the beginning of the next session the client reports that the last session had been very tiring, and the sadness had stayed with her for a few days. But she also reports: "I have gained more space in my body. My shoulders are more open, something is shifting. I can take my space." The therapist writes down these sentences on a piece of paper. She will be giving the client the paper at the end of the session. However, when asked how Vera feels, the client answers: "Vera is not really well yet." Therapist: "Is this an issue for our session today? Or do you need something empowering today? What is your wish?" Client: "I'd like to be in good contact with myself and be able to be loving with myself." Therefore, the therapist decides to instruct the client with the Somatic Experiencing® approach to sense into her inner sensations. She also demonstrates to her *pendulation* and circular breathing (Phillips, 2007), both of which the client can apply at home.

I shall return to the case in Chapter 4 in the section "Restoring Violated Boundaries." There you can also see that with clients who have been parentified, having to take care of a weak or suffering parent, it often is not enough, when only the child ego state has a corrective experience. In fact, the parent part also needs to be taken care of and to feel secure so the child, in this case "Vera," can be discharged and relieved of any responsibility for good.

Overview of the main criteria of a successful (trauma) therapy:

1. Establishing relationship through social support
2. Self-regulation by regulating the basic rhythms in the body
3. Co-regulation in contact with another person

Finding One's Balance

Handling Resistance: The Window of Tolerance

In trauma therapy, if you want to access a difficult or painful experience, the natural resistance of clients should be respected. Overestimating the actual capacity of the organism can lead to hyperarousal and overwhelm with negative emotions or even dissociation, to freezing with muscular constriction in the whole body, and to sensory and emotional numbness. It is advisable to stay in the client's scope of resiliency, to return to resources, that is, to the counter vortex (Levine, 1997) or, if necessary, to pause and scale down the overwhelming sensations and emotions, making them easy to digest so they can be tolerated and integrated. In Somatic Experiencing® therapy this deceleration and scaling down is called *Titration*, as mentioned earlier.

Instead of exploring the memory in detail, you detect where the activation is densified in the body by tracking the body sensations. This activation is expressed in the symptom, where the energy of the incomplete defense reaction of the traumatic experience is stuck. The art is in bringing the interrupted defense reaction to completion and at the same time dosing these powerful energies, so the organism is not overwhelmed again and does not collapse. Titration is needed. Moreover, you have to keep track of the client's window of tolerance (Siegel, 2007). Within this window of tolerance, the client stays curious and can tolerate a higher level of arousal without becoming frightened.

As a metaphor for the scope of optimal activation, Levine (1997) suggests the model of the river of life: In a natural riverbed there is a certain range for floodwater. Even when a river carries more water after a heavy rain, it still stays within its limits. Only when the water level is too high, does it overflow and flood the area. With the human organism, it is the same. As long as the activation does not exceed arousal tolerance, people can expand and so integrate stressful experiences. If the system is overwhelmed, this signifies danger and the automatic survival patterns kick in.

If the boundaries persist, the dorsal vagus can be contained through the social engagement system, while being touched, in the figurative sense, by the other person, to experience healing transformation.

Shifting into Balance

In the case of shock trauma or another traumatic experience, the river is flooded, the riverbanks ravaged, the dams ruptured, creating a dangerous *trauma vortex* (Levine, 1997).

With breached boundaries, experienced as being life-threatening, people feel defenseless, hypersensitive, and overwhelmed, bordering on decompensating. With rigid behavior they desperately seek safety, at the same time experiencing loss of control: They feel overwhelmed and incapable of protecting their boundaries or respecting those of others.

If therapist and client approach the trauma vortex carelessly, they both are pulled into the suction.

Fortunately, there is always a *counter vortex* in the backwater. This, for Levine, is a resourceful counterbalance, a positive, nurturing experience, in which sufferers can find shelter and protective boundaries that are still intact.

Along the lines of the river metaphor, Levine suggests *pendulation* (Levine, 2015) of the attention focus between consolidating and stressful material (see Chapter 8), where you pendulate on the sensory level of somatic sensations between two types of experiential qualities. Not before the client has activated and holds in store a resource that is as contrary to the symptoms as possible and can be felt physically, do you focus on symptoms such as fear, panic, pain, helplessness, shame, physical freezing, or shock. So first, pleasant sensations such as joy, power, warmth, lightness, energy, and the associated sensations are explored and localized, and only then does the therapist invite the client to notice the symptoms, to describe the body sensations associated with them, not longer than is easily tolerable for the client. Subsequently, the focus is directed alternately between the resource and the symptom, thus pendulating carefully between the trauma vortex and the counter vortex. By gently pendulating between these two poles, the unpleasant can be more and more tolerated and loses intensity, symptoms lessen or disappear altogether, and there is a new psychosomatic balance. Therapists accompany the process mindfully and make sure that clients do not stay too long at the edge of a trauma vortex and in no way are seized by the suction attempting to pull them into its depth. If required, the process must be slowed down or even stopped, so that the whole range of the experience can be felt and sensed. Clients are encouraged to notice body sensations, images, emotions, memories, or thoughts coming up spontaneously, and to name them. The exact instructions for pendulation are presented in Chapter 8.

Pendulation is not limited to body sensations, but is possible and helpful on all levels to prevent being sucked into the trauma vortex. Clients can be instructed to pendulate between stressful and resourceful thoughts or between frightening and safety-giving imaginations; likewise, counter vortices can be found on the levels of feelings, sounds, smells, tastes, or touches. Experiencing the concurrence of both poles, as well as the possibility of refocusing and moving back and forth, increases self-efficacy and control, allowing the organism to settle.

In Somatic Experiencing® therapy, during the exploration of symptom-related body sensations, clients are asked about possible movement impulses spontaneously emerging as micro movements or sensed by them.

These movements are then to be executed *slowly*, in *slow motion*, carefully accompanied by the therapist and supported, or restricted, if necessary. At the same time, titrating is important – pausing and sensing into body sensations, as described in the section on Focusing. "What is it like now?" This is all about the body now gradually integrating at its own pace all that was affecting it in such a complex and quick way, that it was not able to react to adequately at the time, so that now it is able to complete the disrupted defense reactions and there can also be a corrective experience on a physical level.

In this process, body-psychotherapeutic methods practiced beforehand, such as breathing techniques, grounding exercises, and other self-regulatory techniques presented in Chapter 8, are helpful. The Voo sound according to Levine is very effective (Levine, Porges, & Phillips, 2015).

In the course of these somatosensory processes, the SIBAM model already mentioned will be useful (Levine, 1991, 2010, 2015) in order to integrate all five dimensions of experience as much as possible. The last stage, the "aha moment," an understanding where the meaning is renegotiated, emerges spontaneously from the present (body) experience as an understanding realization. These are new insights full of content, from which resourceful beliefs develop, as described in the previous case excerpt. Such a result would not be possible through mere reflection.

When the body comes out of freeze and starts moving, the sympathetic nervous system is activated. By physically executing and completing the flight or fight movements in a controlled way, clients find their strength and feel their power again, experiencing a feeling of safety, and the ventral vagal circuit, and with it the social engagement system, are activated again.

Late Triumph: He who Laughs Last . . .

As we have seen, body-based therapy approaches are about creating corrective experiences by resolving, completing, controlling, and coping.

Thanks to humans' imagination and their ability to experience, a threatening situation can be successfully managed even years later and experienced physically as though "happening now." Even a virtual victory can be experienced intensely as gratification. This can have a healing effect on a neurobiological level, because the nervous system is balanced optimally. It is possible to renegotiate the trauma, without necessarily remembering the traumatic content. When fight and flight behavior is completed in a good way, this allows the client to disengage from a defensive orientation and to overview the situation with a newly reclaimed freedom and dignity, orienting more in a curious than a frightened way. Basically, history is being rewritten in the body and on the inner stage when using Ego State therapy. This is more than experiencing something just in one's fantasy, because with the inner stage, inner sensation and emotions change too. Thus, before intervening, an ego state therapist will explain to the client: "You cannot change what has happened, yet you can change how you feel about it inside. You can find inner peace and quiet." This also leads to a "correction" on the inner stage, whereby, in addition to the therapeutic relationship, alliances on all levels play an important role. Such alliances take shape between the therapist and ego states, between the client and ego states, and among different ego states. A safe, coregulating relationship of the therapist with destructive ego states is necessary so they can be integrated supportively into the whole personality. Then, the previously fragmented traumatic memory can finally be memorized in the hippocampus in its entirety, losing its terrifying quality and fading over the years. Curiosity, paired with mental flexibility, is a sign that balance has been restored in the organism and the person can reorient again.

Summary of Somatic Experiencing®:

- Expansion: Through somatosensory experience, focusing on body sensations
- SIBAM: Integrating all relevant "perceptual and sensory channels," thus re-aligning the three nervous systems (ventral vagus, sympathetic, and dorsal vagus) and the three brains (neocortex, midbrain, and brainstem)
- Distancing: Clients are encouraged to be slow and to take charge, by finding *their* rhythm, their pace, and remaining within their window of tolerance. Controlled acting out or imagining mobilization: By spontaneously executing surfacing micro movements in slow motion, fight (pushing, hitting) or flight movements (running, escaping) are completed and thus muscular constrictions are released
- Coming out of a freeze state by focusing on the constriction or using pendulation: Fear is uncoupled from immobility by carefully titrating (helpful to complement with Ego State therapy). Caution: When clients come out of freeze, they are reconnected with their pain or other

unpleasant sensations, and that can be associated with high arousal. Activation of the sympathetic (fight/flight) mode
- Titrating: Granting time and pausing over and over to notice sensory-motor experience. The slower the controlled release, the safer
- Uncoupling: Fear and immobility or anger and helplessness are differentiated through titration and reframing, thus detaching it from the original experience. Consequently, they can be integrated as meaningful survival strategies and experienced as strengths

Notes

1 The more anointing (eye-catching) a stimulus is, the more likely it is to attract attention.
2 In the case of rape, 70 percent of women surveyed who subsequently visited a hospital emergency department responded with tonic immobility, which later correlated significantly with the development of posttraumatic stress disorder (Möller et al., 2017).
3 In the final chapter of this book, suggestions for mindfulness-based body exercises are provided.
4 For example, by Barrabasz et al., 2013, with war veterans.
5 To clarify, MacLean's model is a simplification of the brain that doesn't address more complex functions, many of which are still a mystery. The brain is adaptive. And, of course, new brain structures were not just "added" during evolution. Therefore, MacLean's model has been criticized and rejected by neurobiologists. Nevertheless, the model helps us understand human (emotional) behavior and the effect of trauma and is therefore still useful from a psychological perspective.

References

Barabasz, A., M. Barabasz, C. Christensen, B. French, & J. G. Watkins (2013): Efficacy of single-session abreactive ego state therapy for combat stress injury, PTSD and ASD. *International Journal of Clinical Experimental Hypnosis, 61(1)*: 1–19. DOI: 10.1080/00207144.2013.729377
Beaulieu, D. (2016): *Impact Techniques for Therapists.* Taylor & Francis Ltd.
Csikszentmihalyi. M. (2010): *Das Geheimnis des Glücks.* Stuttgart: Klett-Cotta.
Damasio, A. (2021): *Feeling and Knowing. Making Minds Conscious.* New York: Pantheon Books.
Dilling, H., W. Mombour, & M. H. Schmidt (eds) (2000): *Internationale Klassifikation psychischer Störungen. ICD-10, Kap. V (F). Klinisch-diagnostische Leitlinien.* Bern: Hans Huber.
Eagleman, D. M. (2008): Human Time Perception and its Illusions. *Current Opinion in Neurobiology, 18(2)*: 131–136. DOI: 10.1016/j.conb.2008.06.002.
Emerson, D. & E. Hopper (2014): *Trauma-Yoga. Heilung durch sorgsame Körperarbeit.* Lichtenau: G. P. Probst.
Gendlin, E. T. (2003): *Focusing. How to Get Direct Access to your Body's Knowledge.* Revised and updated 25th anniversary edition. E-Book. London: Random House.
Gordon, I., O. Zagoory-Sharon, J. F. Leckman, & R. Feldman (2010): Oxytocin and the Development of Parenting in Humans. *Biological Psychiatry, 68(4)*: 377–382.
Herman, J. (2003): *Die Narben der Gewalt. Traumatische Erfahrungen verstehen und überwinden.* Paderborn: Junfermann.

Ijzendoorn, M. H. & M. J. Bakermans-Kranenburg (2015): The Role of Oxytocin in Parenting and as Augmentative Pharmacotherapy: Critical Issues and Bold Conjectures. *Journal of Neuroendocrinology, 61*: 2–2.

Klarer, M., Arnold, M., Günther, L., Winter, C., Langhans, W., &Meyer, U. (2014): Gut Vagal Afferents Differentially Modulate Innate Anxiety and Learned Fear. *The Journal of Neuroscience, 34(21)*: 7067–7076.

Levine, P. (2015): *Trauma and Memory: Brain and Body in a Search for the Living Past: A Practical Guide for Understanding and Working with Traumatic Memory.* North Atlantic Books U.S.

Levine, P. (2011): *Somatic Experiencing®.* Training Manual 1st–3rd year in German. Zurich.

Levine, P. (2010): *In an Unspoken Voice: How the Body Releases Trauma and Restores Goodness.* Berkeley: North Atlantic Books.

Levine, P. (1997): *Waking the Tiger – Healing Trauma.* Berkeley: North Atlantic Books.

Levine, P. (1991): The Body as Healer. A Revisioning of Trauma and Anxiety. In: M. Sheets-Johnstone (ed.): *Giving the Body its Due.* New York: State University of New York.

Levine, P., Porges, S., & Phillips, M. (2015): *Healing Trauma and Pain Through Polyvagal Science*: E-Book. www.maggiephillipsphd.com.

Lischke, A., C. Berger, K. Prehn, M. Heinrichs, S. C. Herpertz, & G. Domes (2012): Intranasal Oxytocin Enhances Emotion Recognition from Dynamic Facial Expressions and Leaves Eye-gaze Unaffected. *Psychneuroenocrinology, 37(4)*: 475–481.

Mittag, J., Lyons, D. J., Sällström, J., Vujovic, M., Dudazy-Gralla, S., Warner, A., Wallis, K., Alkemade, A., Nordström, K., Monyer, H., Broberger, C., Arner, A., & Vennström, B. (2013): Thyroid Hormone is Required for Hypothalamic Neurons Regulating Cardiovascular Functions. *The Journal of Clinical Investigations*, 123(1): 509–516.

Möller, A., H. P. Söndergaard, & L. Helström (2017): Tonic immobility during sexual assault – A common reaction predicting post-traumatic stress disorder and severe depression. *Acta Obstetricia et Gynecologica Scandinavia*, 96(8): 932–938. DOI: I0.IIII/aogs.13174 (EPub).

Ogden, P., K. Minton, & C. Pain (2006): *Trauma and the Body: A Sensorimotor Approach to Psychotherapy.* W. W. Norton & Company.

Paulsen, S. (2009): *Looking Through the Eyes of Trauma and Dissociation. An Illustrated Guide for EMDR Therapists and Clients.* BookSurge Publishing.

Phillips, M. (2016): *How to Heal Trauma and Pain Through the Body: Somatic Psychotherapy Level 3*, (Seminar in Zurich, 30 September–1 October 2016).

Phillips, M. (2014): *Somatic Experiencing for Psychotherapists who Work with Trauma &/ or Ego State Therapy, Level 1* (Seminar in Zurich, 16–17 May 2014).

Phillips, M. (2007): *Reversing Chronic Pain: A 10-Point All-Natural Plan for Lasting Relief.* North Atlantic Books U.S.

Phillips, M. & Frederick, C. (1995): *Healing the Divided Self. Clinical and Ericksonian Hypnotherapy: Clinical and Ericksonian Hypnotherapy for Dissociative Conditions.* W.W. Norton & Company, Inc.

Pollak, S. D., Cicchetti, D., Hornung, K., & Reed, A. (2000): Recognizing Emotion in Faces: Developmental Effects of Child Abuse and Neglect. *Developmental Psychology, 36(5)*: 679.

Porges, S. W. (2022): Polyvagal Theory: A Science of Safety. *Frontiers in Integrative Neuroscience*, May 2022, Volume 16. Open Access: Front. Integr. Neurosci. 16:871227. doi: 10.3389/fnint.2022.871227

Porges, S. W. (2017): *Die Polyvagal-Theorie und die Suche nach Sicherheit.* Lichtenau/Westfalen: G.P. Probst.

Porges, S. W. (2015a): *Play as a Neural Exercise: Insights from the Polyvagal Theory.* Porges-play-neural-exercise.pdf [10 May 2018]

Porges, S.W. (2015b): Making the World Safe for Our Children: Down-regulating Defence and Up-regulating Social Engagement to "Optimize" the Human Experience. *Children Australia*, 40(2): 114–123.

Porges, S. W. (2009): The Polyvagal Theory: New Insights into Adaptive Reactions of the Autonomic Nervous System. *Cleveland Clinic Journal of Medicine, 76(2)*: 86–89.

Porges, S. W. (1995): Orienting in a Defensive World: Mammalian Modifications of our Evolutionary Heritage. A Polyvagal Theory. *Psychophysiology, 32(4)*: 301–318.

Ritz, P. (2017): Focusing mit traumatisierten Patientinnen in der Personzentrierten Psychotherapie. *Person: Internationale Zeitschrift für Personzentrierte und Experienzielle Psychotherapie und Beratung, 21(2)*: 132–140.

Sack, M. (2010): *Schonende Traumatherapie: Ressourcenorientierte Behandlung von Traumafolgestörungen.* Stuttgart: Schattauer.

Siegel, D. J. (2007): *The Mindful Brain. Reflection and Attunement in the Cultivation of Well-Being.* W.W. Norton & Company.

Strüber, N. (2016): *Die erste Bindung. Wie Eltern die Entwicklung des kindlichen Gehirns prägen.* Stuttgart: Klett-Cotta.

van der Kolk, B. (2015): *The Body Keeps the Score: Brain, Mind, and Body in the Healing of Trauma.* Penguin LL US.

Chapter 3

The Advantages of
Ego State Therapy

A Relational Therapy

Forming Reliable Alliances

*Ego State therapy helps me understand the background of my compulsions and fears,
and thus to react to the needs of the relevant parts. Engaging with my ego states, I am
learning a new form of "self-empathy."*

(25-year-old client)

Ego State therapy is a *relational therapy*. In contrast to NLP, Gestalt, or other
therapies working with parts, it engages several relational levels at the same time.

By building reliable relationships – between the client and the therapist; between
the client and their ego states; between the different ego states of the client; and
between the therapist and the ego states of the client – not only is it possible to
heal attachment trauma, but also to correct physically and on the inner stage early
traumatic experiences, by using a somatic approach when working with preverbal
parts, allowing for re-enactment and a new experience of these parts. Even though
the past or what happened in the past cannot be changed, it is still possible to neu-
tralize unpleasant or overwhelming emotions associated with experiences made
earlier, to gain distance, to calm them permanently, shifting how one feels inside,
so that the past is no longer terrifying. Intrapsychic conflicts can also be resolved
by identifying the parts involved, hearing and understanding them, and by seeking
a solution together with them. This is done by getting to know each ego state respectfully, listening to them, understanding and acknowledging them, and exploring
their needs before finding out together with them how they can be satisfied.

Growth Thanks to Cooperation

Ego states can *learn, grow, and change*. They *all want to be loved and appreciated*. If you promise them that they will be respected and liked by the clients and
the other parts for what they do, they are also ready to change their role and take

DOI: 10.4324/9781003460602-4

on a new, more sensible function, appropriate in the present moment (Watkins & Watkins, 1997).

Often the different parts do not have the same information. By getting to know each other and sharing, the conflicting parties find more ease with one another and, with the support of the other ego states and the therapist, they can be convinced to collaborate. This results not only in communication but also cooperation among the different parts, experienced by clients as a great relief and as inner relaxation.

This lens is not entirely new, of course, and can be found in other approaches working with parts, as well as in hypnotherapy or Gestalt therapy. However, what is unique to Ego State therapy and its theory is how it deals with sabotaging, destructive parts. These parts are not only externalized, establishing distance from them, but they are also brought in and then utilized. *It would be such a pity to waste or lose the mostly very powerful energy of these ego states!* They actually often become very powerful inner helpers – because these parts originally came to help.

However, they often remain in the past situation, holding onto the strategy originally chosen and do not realize that the individual has advanced and changed since then, and that in the present, other forms of support are necessary.

As soon as they understand that they are still needed and that another form of support would make much more sense at this point, these parts can better grasp ways to both update their notion of support and comply with their original function to help. Knowing that they will be appreciated instead of rejected or even hated, they open to developing new strategies, taking on new tasks that are useful to the client in the present. The ego states acting destructively, once dreaded by clients and therapists, become important supporters and help to promote rather than impede the healing process.

The Corrective Experience in Ego State Therapy

In Somatic Experiencing® trauma healing *and* in Ego State therapy, the corrective experience is of vital importance. It must be experienced. It is not enough to talk about it, rather the client must experience something new and corrective, as described earlier. We know from trauma research, that spontaneous self-healing happens more easily the more resilience there is and the more resources there are. Resilience involves many factors interacting, is rooted in childhood, and is influenced by reactions and is the result of actions later in life. Using Ego State therapy, we now have the possibility to heal wounds, to make up for what was missed out on and thus build resilience through corrective experiences happening on the inner stage and experienced by clients in the here-and-now. Corrective experiences such as these are also possible on a physical level with somatic approaches, breathing techniques, or tapping. They can also occur by "establishing" stable intrapsychic alliances, such as by creating ideal parents who are nourishing, give security, and are always present retroactively, when they are needed (effectively, they do not exist). In this way, parents permanently take care of the child parts, as in the case described with the 40-year-old client in Chapter 2. So, corrective experience is always about *promoting partnerships* and developing strategies together with the clients, especially when therapy is stagnating. Attachment traumata can thus be corrected and healed enlisting reliable, congruent experiences in a safe therapeutic context.

Ego States that Act Destructively

Therapists must always keep in mind that all ego states want to help and be loved, so they not only work with the resource states but also with the unloved ones by trying to understand what their actual and original function – the positive intention – is. That is often very complex, difficult, and lengthy, because these ego states that act destructively not only frighten the client but also the therapist due to their destructive power (for example, massive self-harm or a suicidal tendency). So, one needs to build a therapeutic alliance with these unpleasant, disruptive, or even frightening ego states by determining common goals. If one succeeds in establishing a solid attachment to these unloved or destructively acting parts, enlisting their help becomes possible. In the process, one needs to keep in mind that especially childlike, young ego states are often terribly frightened by these destructive parts. In these cases, it is difficult, yet important, to also bring the parts closer to each other. For if one manages to establish a therapeutic alliance with the parts that are acting destructively, a transformation can take place and they can become a healing energy.

A 62-year-old client with complex trauma, an early attachment disorder, and long-standing experience in psychoanalysis wants to alleviate his depression and anxiety states. The first sessions include self-regulation, strengthening of resources – "What has helped you come out of your panic state?" "When in your everyday life is it the way you would always like it to be?" – psychoeducation, and empowering a two-year-old abandoned ego state. Afterwards, the client is surprised by how clearly the anxiety states and depressive moods have decreased. However, establishing a "safe place" in the fourth therapy session proves to be very difficult. It is not possible to make the place completely safe, as destructive intrusive images or thoughts keep barging in.

In the next session the client reports that his mood has become worse. The panic states and the depression having become much stronger, and that he has been struggling to stay in his adult state and not to fall into childlike panic and helplessness. He could not indulge in such a "safe haven," for as soon as he would withdraw into such a place of security, he would hear "voices" banning him from them. The therapist mirrors these destructive intrusions already surfacing in the very first sessions: "Every time you experience something empowering, these voices interfere. This seems to be an important part that keeps showing up. It certainly is worth getting to know them better, but all in good time. Often such parts develop in traumatic situations to secure survival, as paradoxical as this might seem now to you. But we can find out later." Furthermore, she informs the client about the psycho-physiological processes associated with fear and panic, and about how important it is to focus on the present rather than on the past (trauma) or future (being frightened about future situations). She helps him develop "counter thoughts" and "counter images" to the terror, and she motivates him to practice refocusing on beneficial, opposite images or thoughts as a kind of mental coaching, stepping out of the vicious circle of fear and depression. Then she asks: "How old is the part of you that is panicking?" It is the two-year-old, who is not enough empowered and safe. In addition, the destructive voices keep coming forward.

Because the therapist has the stabilization and empowerment of the entire personality in mind, she shows the client the "over-energy correction" to improve his self-regulation competency and other possibilities of strengthening resources like the "joy journal," before communicating indirectly about the client with the two-year-old and the voices, addressing the adult client in the present to strengthen his "wholeness," the entire personality (and not fragmentation). She explores with him, as the "expert for himself," from an observer's position what the two-year-old needs so he can understand that it is over and he can now have what he had always needed. At the same time, the therapist communicates to the voices that she knows they are important for the client and that she would wish they could cooperate with the other parts in the future and be appreciated by the others, even if it is too early for that right now. Subsequently, the client is relieved, gaining hope again that all will be well. However, another two sessions are needed for the two-year-old to be really reassured and arrive in the present ("that's a nice feeling, moving"), and for the voices to be ready to think about how they could support the client in the future. In addition, it remains important to accompany him with issues of everyday life, self-regulation, the daily practice of self-acceptance, as well as the integration of other injured parts. The therapist talks to the voices again and again to strengthen the alliance. By understanding or meeting the client with his needs and appreciating him and his ego states, a relationship to all of them can be gradually built and the stage is set for mutual understanding, communication, and ultimately, for cooperation. In the section on "Fear and Panic of Traumatized Ego States" in Chapter 4, the work with the "voices" is continued.

This case excerpt illustrates the struggle for stability and safety which, in clients with a history of violence and neglect, can only happen in very small and cautious steps, and it shows how much perseverance is needed from therapists to continue providing safety for the clients and all their ego states without wavering. Yet it also shows that small steps are indeed possible, even if they do not happen straightaway.

Psychoeducating the client regarding fear and trauma is of vital importance. Clients are quite amazed at first, then relieved, when they hear that their body wanted and wants to *protect* them, and that their reactions in light of the threats they experienced are absolutely *normal*. With this information, an actual *reframing* happens. Also, it becomes clear how important it is that the client can keep control and remain anchored in the here-and-now, and how vital self-regulation skills are. Ambivalence and mistrust on the part of the clients are seen as absolutely normal and reframed as important defense and self-assertion mechanisms. They have the possibility of pendulating between trauma and counter vortex, and the more they are in contact with their strengths the better. Moreover, the clients and their ego states have "all the time in the world," nothing has to be rushed. At the same time, hope is sowed time and again, psychoeducation and teaching self-regulation being important conditions.

The case excerpt just presented also shows how the issue can be accessed from many layers, from all sides, based in this holistic approach, and how the therapist has to keep making decisions as to which one of all the possible ways towards integration they want to pursue. In such situations, clients can also always be called in as "experts": "Who should we tend to first? The little one or the voices? What is more important right now? You know best!"

When therapists proceed in this gentle and holistic way and clients become more stable and trusting in the therapy, given the many corrective experiences they and their ego states have, their window of tolerance and resilience will gradually and steadily increase.

Another therapy session illustrates contacting ego states that act destructively:

A 25-year-old student, Manuel, is suffering from compulsive thinking and acting. These were gradually reduced in the course of therapy. His current problem: He is always working. He can hardly sleep at night. He is under a huge pressure, always looking for opportunities to continue writing his papers. He feels this pressure from his neck to his heart region as a "fiery column," unsettling him. On this column, a clock is ticking, running too fast.

Therapist:	What shall I call this part?
Client:	Too-late.
Therapist:	May I speak to Too-late directly?
Client:	Yes.
Therapist *to Too-late:*	Why is the clock running?

Client (as Too-late):	With his two courses of studies, Manuel has a lot to cope with. I remind him that time is expiring.
Therapist:	Since when have you been with him?
Client (as Too-late):	Since he has been at university, for six years.

The therapist explains to Too-late and the client that the organism is much more productive if it can recover and relax once in a while, describing the associated neurophysiological processes with vivid examples, whereupon the client says he actually wished he could have such beneficial breaks but was feeling at the mercy of Too-late.

Therapist:	Is there a part who could provide relaxation? Are there moments of relaxation in your life?
Client:	Yes, very rarely.
Therapist:	How does that feel?
Client:	There is a positive emptiness in my mind. The breathing is less shallow.

The therapist gives the client a bit more time to experience this state more intensely.

Therapist:	What may I call this state with an empty mind and a deeper breathing?
Client:	Silence.

The therapist speaks to Silence, with the consent of the client.

Client as Silence:	Manuel says that relaxation is not okay. He says there is no time for relaxation.
Therapist:	(to the client) Is that right? Is that what you say?
Client:	Yes. It is never good enough. Never perfect!

While talking, his facial expression turns rigid, his voice changes slightly, becoming tighter and more assertive.

Therapist:	Ah, somebody is coming forward for whom it is important that Manuel does everything perfectly! Am I right in assuming that you are the Perfectionist? (This ego state is known from previous sessions.) The client nods.
Therapist	(to Perfectionist): Perfectionist, that is wonderful, that you encourage Manuel to deliver top performances. The problem is only that he doesn't really feel good with that, he is stressed.

Client as Perfectionist:	I don't really like Manuel. I don't care how he feels.
Therapist:	Why?
Client as Perfectionist:	Manuel never does anything right. You have to punish him!
Therapist:	You want to punish him? Why?
Client as Perfectionist:	Actually, he shouldn't even be here!
Therapist:	Why not?
Client as Perfectionist:	It's his fault that his (older) brother hassled him!
Therapist:	I'm sorry you think that, Perfectionist. However, a small child is never to be blamed or held responsible for being abused. The child cannot be responsible, and it is not his job to take care of older siblings or parents, because he depends on them. In fact, like any child, Manuel deserved to not only have been protected back then, but also loved and his boundaries respected. For various reasons this obviously was not the case. And I am sorry. I'm glad that Manuel no longer has to be in this dreadful situation (the little traumatized Manuel ego state was already brought into the present, empowered and integrated in an earlier therapy session). You know, Perfectionist, that you have the same body as Manuel – that you share a body? If you continue to mistreat and punish him, Manuel will eventually break down and you with him!

Perfectionist reacts with confusion.

Therapist:	It would be ideal for both of you if you continue supporting Manuel, but in a way that is good for both of you. Then you would also get more appreciation from him. Teamwork with other parts would be even better. Then Manuel could achieve more and you would all feel better.

After discussing this for a while, Perfectionist is prepared to think about it all until the next session.

Therapist:	Manuel, I am now talking to you again, the adult sitting opposite me. Did you listen? How is that for you now?
Client:	I'm sad. After all, striving for perfectionism was something positive!

The therapist explains to him that striving for perfection can continue but not under the rule of punishing authorities, that is, conflicting parts harming him, but rather with all ego states pulling together, so they can achieve much more, alongside with the inner peace he can gain.

After that session the client feels very good. In the following session Manuel, in a light trance, gathers Too-late, silence and Perfectionist, introducing them to one other, while the therapist suggests exemplary sentences which he uses to make sentences in his own words: "Too-late wants to make amends as much as possible, silence provides relaxation. Perfectionist helped us survive and makes for top performances."

Therapist: It is now becoming clear that you all wanted to protect or help Manuel in your very own way. It's wonderful that you have gotten acquainted with each other. Maybe you can now team up and support Manuel as a team? Today's grown-up Manuel needs your support, for all suffering Manuels are now in a safe place. They can now dedicate themselves to their actual task and support today's Manuel as a team! Together they are much stronger! And is it not promising to be appreciated and respected by the other parts instead of being antagonized? But there is still time for that. Manuel, tell your team what you want.

Client: I want you all to help me in a way that is right for me today.

All states agree.

When asked by the therapist what he still needs, the Client answers, they (his team) need to negotiate some more, they still need time.

Therapist: Let them take their time. I now thank the whole team for cooperating and say goodbye. Manuel, what do you need to complete this?

The client would like to go to his place of wellbeing before reorienting, in order to get a fresh supply of safety.

In the following session, Manuel reports that he had been well, that it had been the first time in a long while that he had not worked on two weekends, and it had been easy for him. He had also noticed that not doing anything had done him good.

This extract from therapy shows how much powerful and punishing ego states are trapped in their role as "lone warriors" and how rigid they are in following and defending it. Often, they do not even know about the existence of other ego states or only notice them vaguely as an oppositional energy. Or they are convinced that the client is still a child and that therefore they have to continue taking on the role that was so vital in the past. Because, in this case, the client had already done a good amount of preliminary work, and some ego states were already known, and the client was familiar with this way of working, quite a lot could be achieved in one session. Here is a basic template for interacting with clients' challenging parts. Keep in mind that some of the steps in the sequences will take longer than others, and that you may have to return to one or other steps to reestablish the contact. The process is necessarily incremental.

More helpful questions:

Do all parts of you agree with this therapy?

What does each ego state need that it does not have yet?

What do you know about the part of you that survived that?

What do you know about a part of you that helps you with . . . (e.g., your fears, your pain)?

Do you know something about a part responsible for . . . (the symptom)?

Which part of you helps you to have this good feeling?

Do you know a part of yourself that is blocking?

Is there a part that all parts trust?

Possible questions to a blocking ego state:

What are your positive intentions?

Who is your opponent?

How could you pursue your intentions without harming X (the client)? Know that you do share the same body!

Do you know that you have the same body?

What could serve everyone, including you? What, in addition, could bring you more appreciation from the other ego states?

Shall we ask the other parts whether they will appreciate you if you cooperate? (These responses should then be shared with the blocking ego state directly.)

As we have seen, resistance is often caused by protective ego states wanting to prevent an overwhelming suffering part being brought into consciousness, thus protecting the client from the bad feelings. If the therapist creates an alliance with this protective ego state, bringing it in versus keeping it out, the therapeutic process can continue. Emmerson (2014) suggests two courses of action when there is resistance:

The first is to appreciate the blocking state, appreciating it and suggesting it cooperate by asking it to be present and observe what is happening. The therapist might say:

> I can see that there is someone protecting the weak, helpless part (*appreciation*). I would like to thank this protective part. I am sure you have been giving this protection for a long time and that was very helpful. It must be very tiring always having to pay attention and be alert (*esteem*). I am also here to help, and while I am here this would be a good opportunity for you to take a well-deserved break. Of course, you would keep an eye open to make sure that everything is done properly (*suggesting cooperation*).

The second course of action is applied with clients who intellectualize or when the approach just described does not work. Emmerson (2014) points out that ego states are very curious to know what the others think about them. With this second course of action, the blocking ego state is directly brought in. If an intellectual part barges in, the therapist might say:

> The part coming forward now seems to be a good thinker. What may I call you? Is Intellect ok? (If the client does not agree, look for another name.) Intellect, I believe you know this Weak part we have been talking about. What do you think about it? Do you like it or would you rather it would disappear?
>
> After Intellect's reply: Now I'd like to know how Weak part feels about what you have said. Weak part, Intellect just said that . . . What's that like for you? What does that feel like?

With this intervention, "Intellect" gets curious about how the "Weak" part feels after what it has said and so listens without blocking. At the same time, the weak ego state has the opportunity to answer questions directly, being accessed immediately without the interference of the protective part (Emmerson, 2014).

Personality parts acting in a highly destructive and malicious way can often be found in clients with severe dissociation phenomena, not only having a dysfunctional effect on the client, but also jeopardizing or blocking the therapeutic process (Watkins & Watkins, 1984). It is often difficult for the therapist to build a relationship, and to interact respectfully with such an ego state acting maliciously. However, without empathy, a safe, co-regulating relationship cannot be established. Without such a relationship, it is not likely that this ego state would be willing to change and integrate as a helpful ego state in the personality.

The following excerpt of a therapy session shows just how hostile such parts can become.

> The client's facial expression changes abruptly, thrusting his lower jaw forward, the corners of his mouth dropping, suddenly appearing to be dismissive, rigid, strict, and angry. Resentfully, he shouts: "What the heck are you doing here? What is all this good for?!"
>
> The therapist responds: Oh, there's someone who does not at all agree with what is happening right now! I can understand that what we are doing here might seem strange to you. Who are you?

Therapists use the emergence of annoyed, angry, or malicious ego states as an opportunity to address them directly and try to come into contact with them, attempting to meet them where they are. It is helpful to imagine the clients and their ego states as actually being a group of clients all present in the room, because how you communicate and proceed is exactly the same. If, in a group therapy, a resentful or angry member comes forward, the therapist pays attention to this individual, trying to understand them. Though therapists will set boundaries with communication rules and their regulatory attitude, they will also give these members the possibility to express themselves within this context. However, malicious, unpleasant ego states are often simply ignored. The more they feel pushed aside, the more vehemently they will continue to act. If a therapist does not let the hostility of such ego states irritate them, instead bearing in mind that these ego states want to protect and defend, the therapist can meet them more openly and respectfully and build a relationship to them.

Ego states acting destructively – also known as perpetrator, destroyer, persecutor, demon, guardian, malicious ego, or alter ego – are often responsible for actions endangering self or others, massive mood swings, somatic or somatoform dissociation phenomena as well as destabilizing flashbacks. They can threaten clients, therapists and the therapeutic relationship (Frederick, 2016). Normally, clients ask therapists to free them from these meddlers. These destructively acting ego states all have the same function – though they often deny it and emphasize how much they want to destroy – which is to protect the rest of the personality from destabilizing trauma content, especially frightened weak child parts.

Frederick (1996) divided destructively acting ego states into three categories:

a) *Functionaries* have helped the person to survive in the past by taking on the attitude and perspective of the offender for the purpose of adaptation, and they stick to this belief.

b) *Janissaries*[1] can be found in long-term abuse. They identify completely with the offender. These ego states are mostly hidden and operate secretly, by making sure the people affected keep living in fear and terror of the abuser, obeying their implicit or explicit veto from the past. These clients also suffer from considerable commitment phobia regarding their relationship with the therapist and rightly fear to be torn by divided loyalties between therapist and Janissary.

c) *Demons* are psychotic and delusional. They do not remember their original purpose and tend to glorify themselves with inflated super myths.

According to Frederick (2016), successful therapy is only possible if the therapist can establish a safe, interactive and cooperative relationship with these destructively acting ego states. The integration of the personality cannot happen before these destructive parts can connect with the other ego states and the self. Nourishing and compensating for gaps in the development and maturation are necessary retroactive tasks. This is a great challenge for therapists, as these destructive parts are often stuck in an early stage of development and do not possess the ability to symbolize or experience object permanence or consistency (Frederick, 2016). From the perspective of McGilchrist's divided brain (2009, 2018), this signifies that these states are not able to pendulate between the chaotic experience of the right hemisphere and the structured experience of the left hemisphere in order to attain an autonomic balance, allowing for cognitive integration (Phillips, 2016). From the perspective of MacLean's triune brain, this means that these parts cannot connect to the neocortex.

Therapists often fall into the empathy trap and mirror deficits, feeling "incompetent, hopeless, powerless, angry, or even antagonistic towards these states," due to the hostility they exhibit (Frederick, 2016).

Porges (2016) illustrates that therapists exhibiting "unregulated" empathy for the suffering of their clients can bring themselves and the clients into a sympathetic adrenal mode or even into dorsal vagal reactions, making constant compassion impossible. Porges emphasizes that empathy can only be experienced in a ventral vagal mode, a mode requiring safety because only then are the sympathetic defense reactions inhibited (Porges, 2016). With their SARI model, Frederick and Phillips (1995) highlighted the importance of safety and trust in the relationship between therapists and clients (Phillips, 2016).

Frederick suggests observing the following aspects, in addition to creating safety and the necessity for therapists to self-reflect regarding transference and counter transference through supervision.

Goodwill is especially important when dealing with destructively acting ego states, which normally reject therapy and therapists. Therapists can prepare themselves for a session with a difficult client by realizing why these destructively acting ego states behave as they do and by noticing their suffering. Cognitive empathy is a prerequisite for compassion. Recognizing and correcting empathy traps provides another possibility for reaching goodwill and empathy.

Persistent communication is vital in working with these states. "Speaking through" can activate the ventral vagus and thus the *social engagement system* and inform silent destructive ego states about other parts and the "inner family," as well as the meaning of the individual ego states, even when bilateral communication is not yet possible. Frederick emphasizes that when therapists persistently seek to communicate, this correlates with the development of trust and empathy (Frederick, 2016).

Hypnotic strategies, such as ideomotor signals, use the unconscious resources of therapist and client and promote the therapeutic relationship, as the therapist becomes a safe model for compassion with all parts of the inner system.

With all these aspects, it is the perseverance of the therapist that creates a safe base for containment and relationship, ultimately allowing for cooperation with the difficult parts (Phillips, 2016).

Table 3.1 offers a compilation of the basic interventions that are helpful for contacting and relating to destructively acting ego states.

Clients must understand that the perpetrator-related ego state developed in order to make the situation back then more tolerable and predictable, and that, at the time, this was the only possibility to survive. The intrapsychic dilemma of the child between helpless dependency and the ensuing adherence to attachment and the agonizing life of a victim is dealt with through an unresolvable "double bind" (Paulsen, 2009). This leads to a behavioral pattern that cannot end in a good result: You can never do justice to both parts; everything you do is wrong. The individual cannot escape this dilemma because the two parts with opposite beliefs are normally separated by an amnesic barrier, so do not know about the existence of the other.

> *A double bind is an ongoing pattern of behavior in which no outcome is a good one. This can apply to intrapsychic dilemmas and mutually exclusive beliefs in which the child cannot possibly resolve them with his/her available information and state of development.*
>
> (Paulsen, 2009, p. 133)

On one side of the amnesic barrier is the helpless suffering child part, on the other is the perpetrator-related ego state that is convinced it is solely responsible for everything. The latter is connected to the power and control of the perpetrator and is therefore a strong energy, normally unconscious, but with all the more effect. Such ego states prevent, for example, clients telling their story of abuse. Once the people concerned understand that it is over, that this inner perpetrator had to develop in order for them to survive, and now has no power anymore, they can begin to differentiate themselves from the state and its needs, and learn to perceive their own needs, discerning them more and more. They can gradually meet this ego state with understanding and acceptance (not for its destructive action, but for the intention behind to secure survival), and, ideally, it will be possible to find a new task for it, such as a protective function adequate in the present time.

Table 3.1 Communication with destructively acting, protective ego states – helpful interventions (© Silvia Zanotta, 2016, Additions to Peichl, 2013, Paulsen, 2009)

1. **Contacting: Praising strength and autonomy**
   Make sure you talk to the destructively acting ego state according to its age and maturity. "I notice you are important for X [for the client]. You are strong, and an important energy. I'd like to get to know you."

2. **Alliance rather than opposition:**
   "I get a sense that you have been extremely committed to X for a long time, but have you been appreciated by X for your high commitment? Have you received acknowledgment?"

   Or: "I have the impression that you are frustrated. You are committed and apparently are getting little or no appreciation from X. Is that right?" (Showing understanding.)

3. **Pick up apprehensions of the ego states, bring clarity:**
   "Does X want to get rid of you? Do you think that I [the therapist] want to get rid of you? I can assure you that, on the contrary, I'd like to cooperate with you. In no way do I want to do without your power/energy. You are a strong energy, so don't worry that you might become irrelevant."

4. **Plant the idea of change in the future:**
   "I know how important you are for X. I wish that sometime in the future it will be possible for you to support X, so that X loves and appreciates you. And that the other parts of X appreciate and acknowledge you, even if this is not yet possible."

5. **Explore the function. For example, what was the original intention of the threat/destruction?**
   "What would happen if you no longer did your job? (What if the system would no longer obey the abuser?) Or: "You certainly have good reasons for acting this way. When did you join X? What was your original intention?"

Table 3.1 (Continued)

6. **Show understanding, appreciation (this is also psychoeducation for X and other ego states listening):**

   "Fortunately, you were there! You helped X to . . . (survive)!"

7. **Reality check:**

   "Is this apprehension still there *today?*"

   a) Is there still contact to the perpetrator?

   b) If not, does the destructively acting ego state know?

   c) Does the destructively acting ego state have the most up-to-date information? "Do you know how old the client is?"

   "Do you know the date today?" "Do you know that you share the same body with [the client]?" (This is often an important question with destructively acting aggressive or auto-aggressive ego states.)

8. **What other feelings and states are behind the aggressive and powerful façade of the destructively acting ego states?**

   For example, is it pain, exhaustion, loneliness, anger at the perpetrator, at other ego states?

   Appreciating perpetrator parts: "Thank you for identifying with the power outside. By doing so, you saved X's life and helped to have at least some control, and maintain the bond to the perpetrator (e.g., the father) that X depended on."

9. **Only when there is a good therapeutic alliance can the most difficult phase of negotiation – a vision of another future – happen:**

   "What do you need that you do not have yet? What would you wish for?"

   "Even if that is not possible now, I would wish that you could fulfill a function that is adequate today, supporting X in a way that is good for X and for you, better than now." (Planting the seed for possible solutions, for hope.) "With new strategies suitable to the present challenges, you could become the most important support for X."

10. **Facilitating, introducing each other:**

    The therapist tries to initiate a conversation between the destructively acting ego state and the client and the other ego states, first clarifying whether they know each other. Often, they only have an inkling of the other's existence, and then have to be introduced to each other (by the therapist or the client). Then, ego states should talk with each other directly, for example, telling the destructively acting state *directly* that they would like it if it cooperated.

    To the client: "What kind of support would you wish for from this ego state from now on?" Possibly ask other ego states for helpful ideas.

11. **Goal:**

    The destructively acting ego state learns to perform its protective function.

Summary of the Ego State therapy:

- All ego states developed in order to help
- All ego states want to be loved and appreciated
- Not all ego states possess the same knowledge, the same information
- Corrective experiences on the inner stage strengthen the entire personality
- The following ego states consistently disturb/block the therapeutic process if they are not recognized/respected: *Traumatized ego states*, in panic, overwhelmed by intense feelings, *blocking or destructively acting ego states*, because they normally fulfill a protective function. These ego states are "frozen" in the past, and either have wrong assumptions or an incomplete knowledge about the present reality of the client.

Interventions with *destructively acting ego states*:

1. *Separating the function* (survival, securing attachment, protection from helplessness) *from the strategy of the ego states* (inadequate perception, (auto-)aggressive, sabotaging behavior, negative, deprecative beliefs, feelings of guilt)
2. *Separating the needs of the perpetrator* (control, power, satisfaction) *from those of the victim* (survival, attachment, control, protection from powerlessness)
3. Differentiation from "outside" real perpetrator
4. On the inner stage: Separating the perpetrator-related ego states from the victim-related ego states
5. Finding out the different needs of all ego states
6. Developing new adequate strategies

Note

1 The Janissaries were the elite group of the army in the Ottoman Empire. They were bodyguard of the sultan and reached the highest positions in the Ottoman state.

References

Emmerson, G. (2014): *Resource Therapy. The Complete Guide with Case Examples & Transcripts.* Victoria: Old Golden Point.

Frederick, C. (2016): *Beyond Empathy.* The Tree of Compassion with Malevolent Ego States. *American Journal of Clinical Hypnosis, 58*: 331–346.

Frederick, C. (1996): Functionaries, Janissaries and Demons: A Differential Approach to the Management of Malevolent Ego States. *Hypnos, XXIII*: 37–47.

Frederick, C. & Phillips, M. (1995): *Healing the Divided Self. Clinical and Ericksonian Hypnotherapy: Clinical and Ericksonian Hypnotherapy for Dissociative Conditions.* W.W. Norton & Company, Inc.

McGilchrist, I. (2018): *How our Divided Brain Constructs the World.* Routledge.
McGilchrist, I. (2009): *The Master and his Emissary: The Divided Brain and the Making of the Western World.* New Haven, CT: Yale University Press.
Paulsen, S. (2009): *Looking through the Eyes of Trauma and Dissociation. An Illustrated Guide for EMDR Therapists and Clients.* BookSurge Publishing.
Peichl, J. (2013): *Innere Kritiker, Verfolger und Zerstörer. Ein Praxishandbuch für die Arbeit mit Täterintrojekten.* Stuttgart: Klett-Cotta.
Phillips, M. (2016): Commentary on "Beyond Empathy: The Tree of Compassion with Malevolent Ego States" (Frederick, C., 2016). *Ego-State Therapy International Newsletter,* January 2017. www.egostateinternational.com.
Porges, S. W. (2016): *Vagal Pathways: Portals to Compassion.* Unpublished manuscript.
Watkins, J. & Watkins, H. (1997): *Ego States. Theory and Therapy.* W. W. Norton & Company.
Watkins, J. & Watkins. H. (1984). Hazards to the Therapist in the Treatment of Multiple Personalities. In: B. G. Braun (ed.), *Symposium on Multiple Personality, the Psychiatric Clinics of North America, 7*: 69–87.

Chapter **4**

Dissociation and Freeze

Shut-down and dissociated people are not 'in their Bodies,' being . . . nearly un-
able to make real here-and-now contact no matter how hard they try. It is only
when they can first engage their arousal systems (enough to begin to pull them
up, out of immobility and dissociation), and then discharge that activation, that
it becomes physiologically possible to make contact and receive support.

(Levine, 2010, p. 112)

Fear and Panic of Traumatized Ego States

The pinnacle of stabilization, and therefore a precondition for the healing process
in trauma therapy – in addition to self-regulation and working with the destructively acting ego states – is to reassure and empower those parts stuck in the traumatic situation because they are overwhelmed by fear and panic. The goal is to
bring them into the present by making them understand that the traumatic situation
is over. This needs to happen before clients can settle and find inner peace. At the
same time, their window of tolerance gradually increases. The parts of their personality that were overwhelmed encountered a threatening situation and could not
integrate or understand the experience. They are still controlled by the same fear
and panic as in the initial situation and bring these feelings to consciousness when
they are triggered, living with the false assumption that the (life) threatening situation continues to exist, that the scary people or the bad situation from the past still
has power over them, thus interfering with the clients' ability to cope adequately
with the challenges of current life using their adult strategies, sometimes even completely preventing them from doing so.

Also Respecting the Boss

Of course, these suffering younger ego states must be empowered and rescued.
However, there is often also a very strong personality part trying to prevent that
from happening, either because it feels it needs to protect the young part, or as a
matter of loyalty towards the perpetrator, or as a destructive ego state, which is
convinced the frightened part does not deserve better. Such destructive parts can be

DOI: 10.4324/9781003460602-5

internalized perpetrators keeping up the trauma on the inner stage and torturing the child parts, although the real perpetrator no longer has any influence in the outside world and may not even be living anymore. These blocking states are often very powerful in the inner system, controlling the frightened state or states, making the client's life miserable, with self-destructive tendencies or behavior harming others. Therefore, therapists are well-advised not to ignore them, but rather seek to communicate with them. Often you must first tend to the "top boss" (Paulsen, 2009) and bring them in or make them a co-therapist (Emmerson, 2014), before being able to take care of the frightened parts. Otherwise, these parts can sabotage the corrective experience.

Another excerpt from working with the 62-year-old client traumatized by his psychotic mother, described in Chapter 3, is mentioned here as an example.

Following stabilization techniques in the first two sessions (*conflict-free experience*, introducing *inner helpers*, bringing all suffering parts to a safe place, establishing an *inner observer*, *psychoeducation*), unsettling negative images and thoughts, as well as overwhelming fears and panic keep emerging. The therapist encourages the client to allow for the *simultaneity of resource and trauma* so he can try pendulating between the two. The following images appear for the two states: On the one hand, the stormy sea; on the other, the quiet sea. The client remembers music from an English Renaissance sonnet soothing him. In the following session the issue is his enormous fear of abandonment. The therapist asks him to imagine a specific situation in which he was overwhelmed by this fear.

Therapist: What is it like?
Client: They have all forgotten me. I have to gasp for air. I'm not getting what I need!

A two-year-old boy appears, alone in his room, in the dark. The therapist tells him that it is over and he can now change his environment and does not have to be alone in the dark anymore. With the support of the therapist the little one can have a corrective experience, he can be on the lap of a loving mother at the family table. However, deprecatory images and sentences keep surfacing. The little one feels like a scapegoat. Scapegoat, also an infant, is being insulted in a very nasty way by the mother, telling him he is a "filthy demon." After having empowered Scapegoat and brought him back into a safe present, the therapist says: "Now that you have shrunk your mother and she can no longer scare you, you can tell her anything you like. You are now safe, nothing can happen to you."

Client as   Keep your filth to yourself! You don't have any power over me
Scapegoat: anymore!"

With the help of the therapist, a cocoon with a safe boundary is established around Scapegoat. Then she invites him to pass through something cleansing (*separation sieve*). Scapegoat chooses a golden grid, collecting everything he no longer needs or does not want anymore, after which he feels good. "There's much light around me."

Therapist:	Does the name Scapegoat still fit now? No? What shall I call you now?
Client:	Daniel.

Following this intervention, the client remembers another song, which leaves him with much skepticism. These are signs that the corrective experience was not successful or not completed.

After this session, the states of anxiety and depressive mood distinctly diminished. The client is surprised, but while working exclusively with resources in the next therapy session, he is overcome by doubt, and subsequently overwhelmed by panic attacks and intrusive images and thoughts again. Little Daniel is no longer safe and also no longer on mother's lap. There are Voices telling the client, "You shouldn't allow yourself to even exist," as soon as he wants to connect with his resources. The therapist tells the client, at the same time addressing the Voices: "I know that these Voices are important and that originally they also helped you to survive. Maybe they cannot remember anymore and cannot imagine that they could possibly do something other than to punish and debase. But I also realize that they are important. May I speak to the Voices directly?" The client consents.

Therapist to Voices:	I realize that you are important. I'm curious to know you. Do you know how old X is?
Client as Voices:	Two years old.
Therapist:	Oh, okay. Then I understand why you are so vehement. You want the two-year-old to be as invisible as possible so that he is not constantly tortured and abused by his mother. It's a good thing you were there at the time. Now you will hear something that will surprise you: This was over a long time ago, because today he is 62 years old and autonomous. His mother can no longer harm him.

Subsequently, the Voices and the client undergo thorough psychoeducation. The therapist promises them new strategies and approval from the client and the other ego states. They still need time but agree that the therapist and the client can now take care of Daniel. A horse brings him to his "Mother in heaven." There, he is finally safe forever. Little Daniel and the client now also believe it – that is, they have understood that the little one will now always be safe. The therapist shows the client the *over-energy correction* as an additional possibility of self-regulation, to be practiced at home.

In the following sessions, corrective experiences for other young, frightened parts happen, instantly succeeding, because now they are no longer being sabotaged. The Voices gradually turn into a cooperative protective part, Bolted.

Now, a lasting stabilization actually takes place, allowing the fear states to disappear and the depressive moods to gradually subside. Being alone is no longer frightening.

Signs of Ego States in Fear and Panic

If states of fear are not resolved or the frightened ego states are not empowered and integrated, they can make themselves felt with the following symptoms:

Nightmares, insomnia, phobias, panic attacks, various fears, mood swings, a posttraumatic stress syndrome (PTSS), self-harming behavior, generalized fear, dissociative phenomena to the point of a dissociative identity disorder (DID), addictive behavior, compulsive disorders, instability.

In therapy, scared or panicking ego states often surface spontaneously when you explore the situation or behavior the clients want to change, or when the therapist invites the client to describe a specific situation in which the unwanted behavior or feeling occurs.

The procedure with states overwhelmed by fear and panic – Emmerson (2015) calls these states "vaded with fear" – was described in some of the case studies and is specified in Chapter 8, with instructions for two alternatives: 1. *Bringing frightened, powerless ego states into the present*; 2. *Nourishing retroactively, corrective experiences.*

Nightmares

In addition to the hypnotherapeutic method in which you change the action in the dream so that the dream has a happy ending, Ego State therapy offers the possibility of freeing the challenging part(s) causing the fear, defusing them, so that peace can prevail again on the inner stage and the cause of the disturbing dreams can be corrected. As described in the next therapy excerpt, it is not necessary to know the content of the trauma or the specific cause of the dream. In the example, we need not know why "Mini-Julia" feels so lost; rather, it is her reaction to the dreams that is critical and the fact that she can now change it and have a lasting corrective experience.

All of a sudden Julia, 23 years old, is totally unsure, still suffering from a sense of doing everything wrong. She keeps suffering from a recurrent nightmare in which she is being chased and though she tries to wake up from her dream, she cannot. She is terribly frightened by this nightmare.

The therapist lets the client describe the dream in detail. Then she asks about the worst scene. Julia reports that the worst part is being chased. Then the therapist invites Julia to imagine being a script writer able to rewrite the film: I don't know where you would like to start changing your script, your film. Take your time to rewrite your film story so it ends happily . . . You are the scriptwriter; you decide on the story! Julia's first change is to have her friend help her and to arm herself with a shield, armor, and a pistol. In a light trance she plays the new dream in her mind. She is being chased by three men. Instead of running away, she faces them, pulling out her pistol, shield, and armor, yelling at her persecutors to shove off. During this scene, her boyfriend is always behind her to support her. When asked by the therapist how she feels now, she replies: Much safer!

Therapist: Where in your body do you feel that?
Client: From head to toe.
Therapist: What do you need so you can feel 100 percent safe and protected? You know that in your film everything is possible. You decide on what your heroine needs!
Client: A bubble of light is protecting me. (She settles noticeably.) The persecutors are confused . . . I hit them and drive them away!
Therapist: Very good. Great! . . . How does that feel?
Client: Liberating, strong, and free, safe . . . I allowed them to intimidate me . . ., but now I can defend myself.

After a new script full of resources for her dream has been found, the therapist chooses to add ego state work with the part of Julia that is insecure. She asks Julia to imagine a specific situation in which she is overwhelmed by this insecurity, and explores the body sensations associated with it. Mini-Julia appears. She is very small, lost, pressuring herself with expectations towards herself that are too high. What does mini-Julia want? She would like to become big, stand upright, be self-confident, take one day at a time and take it easy.

Therapist to mini-Julia: You can now have all that, in exactly the way adult Julia changes her dream. You now have the power and possibility to change your environment in such a way that you have everything to stand straight, self-assured, and take one day at a time!

Mini-Julia gets big, she is lying on an air bed in the pool, protected by an air bubble. She is very relaxed, wearing sunglasses and enjoying a drink, having a good time. Now, adult Julia feels "quiet and calm."

Preverbal Traumata

The treatment of trauma begins with the basic functions of a body being able to sleep, rest, feel safe and being able to move.

(van der Kolk, 2017)

. . . helping a client recover from developmental trauma is life-changing – not only in this generation, but for future generations as well.

(Kathy Kain & Stephen J. Terrell, 2018)

Signs of Preverbal Trauma

Trauma experts (i.e., van der Kolk, Peichl) have pointed out that when memories on the verbal level or images are missing, there is a high probability that trauma happened at a very early stage in human development, before acquisition of language, and is therefore stored in the implicit sensory "body memory."

With these early traumata, symptoms have existed for a long time, such as (chronic) pain, diffuse or missing body sensations ("not being in one's body"), constrictions in certain parts of the body or feelings of numbness (as though parts of the body were split off), digestive problems (i.e., diarrhea, constipation, or alternating conditions), etc. In therapy, they surface either as states of panic or existential angst with high arousal or as the type of freezing found in dissociation. The client has difficulty speaking, speech is either unemotional or with very little emotion, with no facial expression, body posture seems sunken due to mainly hypotonic musculature (collapse), breathing is shallow, the complexion is pale, the eyes are not focused, there is a high sensitivity to light or sound. The client might be cold all of a sudden or feel nauseous, describing feelings of numbness, rigidity, or tension, as if paralyzed or "frozen." By what means can we reach these largely autonomous states not accessible to awareness? We need methods to contact implicit sensory memories. Here, Somatic Experiencing® trauma therapy offers effective means, especially with the exploration of involuntary movements and slowing titrating them, as well as using pendulation.

The 38-year-old client fell because she fainted during a flu and hurt her foot, triggering early (attachment) traumata as well as a complex pain syndrome, which was treated unsuccessfully when she was between 20 and 30 years old. At the time, she could not walk longer than 30 minutes at a stretch.

Now she does not feel her feet properly, is unsteady on her feet, and wishes her feet could belong to her again. The therapist asks her to describe the fall in detail. It becomes clear that she got away lightly and that her body made sure she only received minor injuries. The therapist explains that to her and emphasizes the difference between this present experience and the earlier traumata.

Therapist: Is there a part or area of your body that feels stable and safe that you can sense well?
Client: Yes, my flanks.
Therapist: Please keep your attention there for a moment. Describe to me what your flanks feel like.
Client: They are warm, strong, firm, and clear. That makes me feel safe.

After a while the therapist asks the client to move her attention to her feet.

Therapist: Try coming into contact with your feet. What's that like?
Client: It is nearly impossible; I only feel part of my feet.
Therapist: Where do you feel them the most?
Client: The best contact is at the soles of my feet.
Therapist: Now contact your right foot. What does it feel like? If it could speak, what might it say?
Client: There is a slight pain from the injury. Since the fainting, it has been like in a state of shock . . . it believes it is a normal foot that can heal itself.
Therapist: I see, that's interesting! And the left foot?
Client: The left foot does not believe that. It is also in a state of shock. Ouch . . . it's like it's thawing after having been frozen, and that hurts!
Therapist: Who can tell the left foot that it is over, in a way it can actually believe it?
Client: The Reasonable One. (The Reasonable One is a state known from previous sessions.)
Client as   It is really over, that was only a memory surfacing. The body
Reasonable: was able to protect itself from the fall, it fell on the right side.
Therapist: How is the left foot reacting? What does it think?
Client: It says, it was a nightmare, but it believes Reasonable.

Therapist:	What is needed now?
Client:	All the terrible years should be washed out of the foot, together with the pain. The pain in the foot should dissolve!
Therapist:	Who might help?
Client:	The dervish (a familiar resource state from an earlier phase of therapy)
Therapist:	How can she help?
Client:	She takes her left foot into her hands; she has an ointment with cinnamon with which she nourishes and tends to her foot. She also makes clear: It is over!

The therapist gives the client time for this process of nourishing and healing.

Therapist:	What is it like now?
Client:	The left foot must recover its dignity. That takes more time.
Therapist:	Maybe you can connect the feet and the flanks in some way, I don't know how . . . with your breath, with your imagination, or just by sensing it . . . so feet and flanks can connect, and so that it gets better for the feet . . .

Again, the therapist gives the client some time.

Therapist:	I would now like to invite you to focus again fully on your feet, being aware of the connection to the floor. What is it like now?
Client:	I feel my feet again, and the connection to the floor. It still takes the healing and nourishing of the Dervish but my feet are firmly on the ground again, the pain is nearly gone.

In the next session, the client reports having felt good and fit again soon afterwards. Since then she has been anointing her feet every evening with the cinnamon balm. This has been healing and pleasant. Yet two more sessions of nourishing are necessary for the feet to become really stable and feel alive and no longer cold.

This therapy excerpt illustrates once more that it is not the content of experienced trauma that is important, but rather the client's reaction to it. The therapist sticks to exploring the client's body sensations and pendulating between the flanks, feeling strong, and the feet that are numb at first, then hurt (left foot), and in the end can be felt again nicely. At the same time, the difference between the past and the present is emphasized over and over, and a familiar resource state is brought in to help. In the context of a corrective experience, renegotiation on the inner stage and on the physical level happens. Moreover, a new meaning is generated with an alliance between the left foot in shock and the strong "dervish," allowing inner conflicts to resolve. In further sessions, cooperation between them is consolidated. It is impressive how the healing impulse surfaces spontaneously, namely the pain growing out of the left foot and the client later embalming it, thus consolidating and anchoring the new experience.

In early trauma, co-regulation (described several times) and teaching and supporting self-regulation are particularly important. As seen in the section on "Pre-verbal Trauma," corrective experiences can happen on different levels, notably with early attachment trauma, with the help of *hypno-somatic or multimodal Ego State therapy*:

• Between the client and the therapist through coherence and containment
• Between the clients and their body through self-regulation and mindful perception of body sensations
• On the inner stage through corrective stable relationship experiences

On the inner stage, very young parts can come into contact with strong states, for example, with ideal parents or inner helpers. When young states can profit from this kind of support they learn to establish safe and empowering connections between each other, so that an inner team can develop and grow. Partnerships between the ego states can be encouraged as support when necessary.

Thus, attachment traumas are healed by creating safe inner bonds. Again, in this context, the connection with the core self is very important (inner strength, inner wisdom, *conflict-free experience*). Moreover, the exercises presented in the last chapter of this book, *Welcome to the World* created by Diane Heller and *Loving Eyes* by Jim Knipe, are useful for planting ideas and examples of safe bonds. Clients with traumatic bonding experiences often have no model for imagining reliable attachment figures, they first must be created. In this phase, concrete suggestions made by the therapist as to how safe attachment works are useful, as are stories in which safe bonds are illustrated alongside the forms they can take. This process gradually allows for corrective experiences to happen, step-by-step.

With early trauma, making up for early developmental deficits plays an important role. Because early trauma often involves the violation of boundaries, it is crucial to establish boundaries and to sense and learn how to self-assert. In addition, frequent inner relationship conflicts, often happening unconsciously, between ego states or between the client and one particular ego state, can finally be resolved.

Developmental delays can often be seen in these clients *and* the traumatized ego states. Therapists must make sure to respect the level of maturity and the (cognitive) abilities of these ego states when contacting them.

The 28-year-old client reports suffering from various fears. Currently, she is learning to drive and suffers from fears when she has made a mistake. Then she thinks: "I will never learn this anyway!"

When asked by the therapist what has helped so far, she answers: "It helps to talk to myself. I kept telling myself: You can do this! Or: Now I'm going to do this!"

The therapist asks the client to imagine a specific situation where this thought of "I can't manage" emerged (*to immerse oneself in a specific situation*).

The client describes the following situation: She is having a driving lesson, nothing works, then the terrible feeling shows up: I can't do this anyway . . .

Therapist:	Where do you feel this? What does that feel like? (*naming associated body sensations*).
Client:	There is a tension . . . a tingling at the side of my arms . . . also a feeling of emptiness and a slight nausea in my belly. If I could, I would leave quickly and just quit. I can't do it anyhow and don't want to do it.

When asked by the therapist to stay with these sensations for a moment, the client says after a while: My arms feel defiant (*pausing, sensing*).

Therapist:	Your arms seem to want to protect you (*active listening*).
Therapist:	What does your belly want to say?
Client as belly:	I believe I can't do it.

With the permission of the client, the therapist speaks directly to the arms: I'm glad that you are protecting the belly. It is terrible to feel you can't do it.

The client now seems completely helpless, collapsed. *Therefore, the therapist asks the client to stand up. She continues to work with the client while she is standing.* She invites the client to choose a place in the room for strength (I can manage!) and weakness/fear (I can't cope!). The therapist asks: Where is the place for strength? What's the place for weakness/fear? Then she asks the client to go to the place of strength first and to stand there (*from freeze to movement*).

Therapist:	What is it like?
Client:	The arms feel strong!
Therapist:	Yes, the arms obviously help to protect. Just feel your arms, let them do what they want to do without thinking.

The client begins making defense movements with her arms, starting gradually to move.

The therapist invites the client to pause, rest, and sense what it is like, repeating the procedure several times.

Client: It feels more calm, there's less tingling . . .

In several steps the client makes the defense movements and then rests and tracks her sensations. (*titration, resolution*).

Therapist: Only you know when it's enough. Take your time.
Client: The tingling is becoming more pleasant. The arms notice that they have strength and that they can use the strength! (*From helplessness to strength*)

The client begins to relax, and there is a slight rocking of the whole body to and fro, more and more into balance.

Client: Now there is a pleasant feeling of weight. There's strength!

Then the therapist asks the client to go to the weak place, into the position of fear: She immediately feels, "all small and weak, unpleasantly empty, below the diaphragm, cold," and she feels nauseous.
    The nausea comes very quickly and vehemently. The client has to sit down.
    The therapist reassures her: That is a terrible feeling, to be so powerless. May I speak to this powerless part?

Therapist: What may I call you?
Client: Little One.
Therapist to This is not happening now, it is over! It is a memory. You are
Little One: safe now. It's over!

Little One calms down. Since the session is coming to an end, the therapist suggests to the client to surround herself with a protective cover.

Client: In here, it is lovely and warm. I do not have to do anything; I have everything I need!

The client relaxes even more. Before completing the session, the therapist asks the client to go back to the place of strength to reconnect to her resources.
    During the short debriefing, the client says she is shocked at how dizzy and nauseous she felt, since she normally does not get those sensations. It had only stopped when the therapist said: It is over!

In this case excerpt, the therapist is assuming that there is a small, young ego state being triggered during the driving lessons, abruptly dampened in its urge to explore and consequently having internalized the belief: I can't do this anyway! In infants, this is often associated with a deep experience of shame, as we will see in Chapter 6 on shame and guilt. When clients fall into these early states, they become immobile or feel nauseous. Therefore, it makes sense to work standing up, as was shown in the previous session, because it is easier for clients to start moving. By shifting her positions, the client was not left in a state of fear for too long.

When treating early trauma, the "five R's," suggested by Phillips (2016), and in Phillips and Frederick (1995) can be used as a structural help:

- *Repair: Facilitating corrective experiences*
- *Renegotiate*
- *Reestablish attachment*
- *Resolve: Resolving conflicts*
- *Reconsolidate and connecting*

In Somatic Ego State therapy, a multimodal approach including the body, *corrective experiences* happen in the therapeutic relationship, the relationship of the clients to themselves, on a body level and on the inner stage, as was just described. *Renegotiating* means slowly approaching the traumatic experiences while at the same time building resources and stability: The clients and their weak ego states are to be *empowered*, resources anchored, facilitating pleasant next to difficult body sensations. Through pendulation, starting with the resources as an anchor, to the less pleasant sensations, clients can be made to feel contraction and expansion. Levine calls this kind of renegotiation a "transformative power." By carefully *identifying* and *observing* the difficult sensations, feelings and images without being overwhelmed by them, there is resolution and integration, memories no longer feeling threatening (Levine, 2015). In this process, clients first have to learn to name sensations and to gradually self-regulate difficult feelings and sensations. In the last chapter, we suggest a collection of possible body sensations that can be offered to clients to help them find words and express what feels appropriate for them. Another possible introduction to pendulating and focusing on the breath and body sensations at the same time, is the *5-minute heart intervention* (Phillips, 2016), also explained in detail in the last chapter.

Something simple to do and surprisingly effective is changing one's posture, similar to the problem and solution choreographies done by Gunther Schmidt (2010). Just by adopting a contrary or completely different body position, the inner feeling also changes abruptly. Clients can try out and practice a suitable body posture together with the therapist. Instructions on how to *change posture* are also given in the Chapter 8.

Often the contact with ego states is easier and more immediate on a body level, and solutions emerge surprisingly quickly. Ego state therapists exploring this are surprised time and again by how easily and quickly changes happen. This is especially found with clients who are very rational and tend to intellectualize, as directing the focus on the body brings ease and spontaneous solutions because they cannot question every step.

Relationships are *repaired* by not only creating the corrective relational experiences mentioned, but also by strengthening the whole personality with breathing and mindfulness exercises, ego state techniques such as "inner strength," "the inner conference room," or the *conflict-free experience* presented in the last chapter. When *resolving inner* conflicts through techniques from Ego State therapy, techniques from the Somatic Experiencing® approach are also used. If there are incomplete or disrupted defense reactions, the sensations associated with them are first explored carefully. In case it is still necessary, the therapist supports the completion of these reactions that are stuck or lets the clients imagine them.

Consolidating and connecting is about strengthening as a focal power in therapy and on all levels. To stabilize the client's personality, it is helpful to use self-hypnosis, a stabilizing trance, writing down new insights and beliefs and practicing self-regulation. If, in addition, a connection to transcendent powers such as angels, fairies, and magicians is made on the inner stage, the probability of containing or neutralizing demons and destroyers is increased.

Utilizing Spiritual Resources

Many people affected by trauma were able to cope with their upsetting experiences thanks to their spiritual resources. It is worth asking the questions:

"How did you survive all this? What helped you?"

Often clients name other people first. However, they must also possess their own resources in order to survive. It is vital for healing to get to know and appreciate these strengths and, if necessary, to reactivate them for the present. Sometimes there are also spiritual ego states such as "Mother Earth" or "Angel Gabriel," especially when their trust in other people has been undermined and no human figures can be imagined when nourishing neglected ego states retroactively. Such spiritual ego states are all-loving and almighty and act as a healing counterpart and opposite image to the upsetting and grim figures or experiences from the past. These personality parts can help create hope and play an important role in trauma healing (Paulsen, 2009).

Reconnecting through Tapping

Tapping techniques are also a possibility of self-regulation and are suitable for finding a way out of freeze, collapse, and dissociation. Tapping directly under the

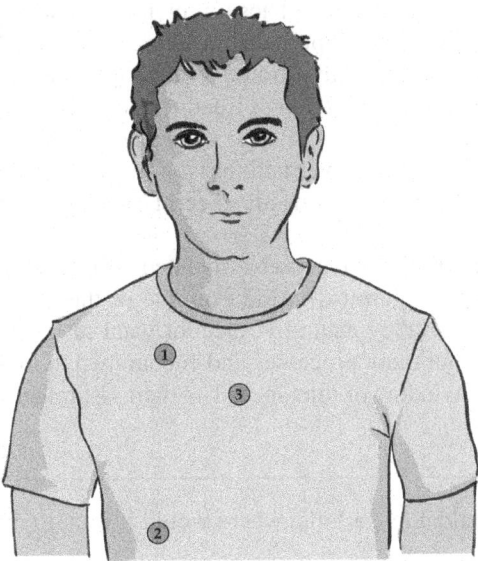

Figure 4.1 Tapping points for freeze, collapse, and dissociation

clavicles, on the sternum, on the two lowest ribs, seems to work best with dissociation, collapse, and freeze. In Figure 4.1, these would be the points 1, 3, and 2.

From Freeze to Mobility

Early trauma and dissociation are inevitably associated with a freeze reaction. Clients instinctively fear activation and arousal and the horror felt at the time of traumatization associated with it. The more distinctively and longer the dissociation exists, the greater this fear. And rightly so. The parasympathetic activated in a dorsal shutdown or collapse inhibits to a great extent the sympathetic activation, namely the fight or flight reaction necessary for defense. The therapist can explain this to the clients (psychoeducation), letting them know that the freeze was the best solution for them *back then*, but that they *now* have other possibilities. If this immense amount of energy was activated for the defense of the organism and then suspended or frozen, both the sympathetic and the parasympathetic branch of the nervous system can be fully activated. It is as though they were stepping on the accelerator and brake at the same time. The sympathetic tries to stimulate the body's resources as a reaction to the threat while, at the same time, the parasympathetic tries to stop the metabolism via the dorsal vagus – creating a physiological dilemma (Levine, 1997). This excessive blocked energy either presents itself as a hyperarousal or as a standstill.

The earlier during the period of physical development the trauma happened, the fewer connections existed between the three brains and the bigger the risk to keep falling into a freeze reaction. These immense physical energies associated with the fear and terror of the experienced trauma should be discharged in small steps, slowed down, and carefully titrated to uncouple the fear from the reaction of immobility. Here, the combination of treatment with Ego State therapy is helpful: By speaking directly through the ego state stuck in the trauma, the therapist can let that part know that it is over and that it now has the ability and possibility to defend itself, as described in various excerpts from case studies presented in this book.

When the protective freeze reaction associated with feelings of numbness dissolves, clients feel pain again (as in the example of the left foot), and other unpleasant feelings, which they naturally reject or want to fend off. Therefore, they must be informed about these processes and encouraged to tolerate the unpleasant feelings within their window of tolerance. The therapist might ask:

"If your body could move a little, where would it want to move?"

In order not to overwhelm clients with the high arousal, and thus re-traumatizing them, this activation can be made tolerable by adding pendulation, slowing down, repeatedly pausing, sensing ("What's it like now?") and grounding or anchoring, and the defense reactions can be completed in a controlled manner. If the body can execute these natural impulses, the tension releases, leading to a huge relief, as illustrated in various case studies.

The physical discharge during the completion of the survival reaction expresses through symptoms such as shaking, trembling, vibrations, goosebumps, and warm sweat. Also possible are autonomic motor reactions that can last several minutes and end in deep breaths such as sighing or yawning, and ensuing relaxation.

The case study with the client "Sandrine" in Chapter 1 shows the titration of high arousal by *calming the breath* and the heartbeat in small steps by *slowing down the hand movement* and by *orienting to the outside*: Look around! Is there something that calms you? After the high arousal, these interventions allow for a deep relaxation of the whole organism.

How creative the human organism is when it comes to problem solving can be seen in the next case study excerpt.

A 48-year-old client complains about various eczema outbreaks, reporting that she always suffers from something that bothers her without knowing what the trigger is. Already as a child her immune system had always been an issue. She would like to stabilize her "center" (back and belly). The therapist asks her to focus completely on her body, noticing what is.

Client: I'm very nervous, I feel fidgety, a kind of "Zzzzzz" on my skin. I feel so insecure, like walking on ice. This city is too dense, too loud, stressful . . . I have to stand up!

She stands up and continues feeling into her sensations: It's so hollow in my belly, it feels like a balloon. At the same time, there is this fidgety feeling in my facial muscles and feet, I feel so wobbly . . . I am nowhere, like a soap bubble, without a core, no weight, like an embryo not having a spine and feelings yet.

She starts making flowing movements, first with her arms, then with her upper body, and finally with her whole body, accompanied by the words of the therapist:

Therapist: Very good. Yes, exactly. Let your body move, very slowly, in slow motion.
Client: I have to explore . . . All my thinking is flowing into this nothingness, there are no stories, emotions, no sensations.

The therapist encourages her to explore more.

Client: Now that is covered by sadness, like a pile of algae.
Therapist: Fortunately, this is over now. You have carried this pile of algae long enough. It is time to get rid of it. You can now liberate yourself from it!

The client stretches, spreading her arms, her graceful movements becoming ever more powerful, and then softer again.

Therapist: What's it like now?
Client: At the back it feels pleasant. I now have support in my back and am able to stand well. Behind, it is darker and more dense – in front, it is brighter.
Therapist: Is the dark pleasant or unpleasant?
Client: It is pleasant, heavy, but pleasant . . . In front, it is light. Am I protected there?
Therapist: Let your body continue exploring.
Client: It feels quite powerful! There is a longing to be so powerful!
Therapist: Yes, exactly. And you know what? From now on you can keep this power!

Client: Something still doesn't believe that.
Therapist: Just let your body take over, trust it!

The client continues with the movements of her arms and trunk that are still gracefully flowing but much more powerful. The therapist accompanies this process by talking to the prenatal part.

Therapist: Enjoy this warm feeling of being secure and looked after. You are being awaited with joy. You keep hearing your mother speak to you, you already know her voice quite well, enjoying when she caresses her belly and is in contact with you. And when it is time and you are ready to go out into the world, then you will be welcomed joyfully by your Mummy and your Daddy. They are crying with happiness and are deeply touched that they can hold you in their arms and caress you. They welcome you and love you unconditionally.

In the following therapy session, the client reports she very much liked coming into this primal state. "It was impressive. It felt good being free without being earthbound. Then, however, there was sadness, the legacy, the coat that I had to put on back then. But I also experienced, this feeling does not belong to me. I can get rid of it."

This session is also about a little child who experienced neglect and rejection, a little one who would like to hide and get away and is frightened. This unloved child is also welcomed, duly appreciated and cherished; tears are shed. After this corrective experience, the client says: I am bigger, everything is clearer. It was never like that when I was a child.

Asking Other States for Help

You can also ask other states for help if you meet a part that cannot yet speak or speaks another language. This situation can occur in an ego state that developed before language acquisition or in an ego state that speaks another language and doesn't understand the therapist's language. The therapist can then ask another ego state, i.e., an observing part, to speak for the preverbal part or to translate for the part that speaks another language. The therapist might say: She (the preverbal ego state) cannot speak yet, do you want to lend her your voice? Or: Is there a part that could translate for her?

The therapist needs to account for either circumstance because the child ego states may not understand or could react with confusion. Generally, it is worth inviting clients speaking another language to say important sentences out loud in their own mother tongue and then feel into the resonance that happens in their body: Is it right like that? Or do you have to rephrase the sentence slightly?

Chantal[1] has forgotten her English mother tongue. She spent the first four years of her life in Australia. Due to her parents' separation, the mother moved to Belgium with her where she was placed in a boarding school with nuns although she did not understand a word of French. Nobody spoke English with her so she learned the French language quickly. For a while, she still dreamt in English. First, the therapist asks for a resource: Chantal feels a fireball in her lower abdomen, seeing magma and a dragon, emanating an enormous power.

Therapist: How can we communicate with the dragon?
Client: We are connected telepathically.

The therapist addresses the dragon directly and asks it what it wants. It would like Chantal to listen more to it, to respect and notice it more.

Therapist: What's that like for you, Chantal?
Client: It gives me life. It's as though I was emerging from a shelter.

Visibly moved, she reports how she is flying with the dragon, being at the same time above it and in it.

Therapist: Where are you flying to?
Client: Into outer space . . . it is beautiful . . . We are witnessing the birth of the planets . . . But there is something that is tensing up, cramping in my feet and legs.
Therapist: Stay with that sensation in the legs for a moment . . . Do you feel movement?
Client: No, it's relaxing . . . I've lost my roots. Instead, I can now fly and the dragon lets me feel its power.
Therapist: If you now think of the sudden move from Australia to Belgium, what do you notice?
Client: Sadness.

After having explored the body sensations associated with it, the therapist asks: How old are you?

Client: I'm four years old. I'm not allowed to cry.
Therapist: That is not okay. Every child has the right to cry whenever it feels like it. Listen, this is not happening now, it is over. You

now have the power to change your environment or to leave. You have the right to be cared for in a language that is familiar to you. Like any child, you deserve to be safe and secure. It is not your fault that you wound up there. You can cry whenever you feel like it. It is not your fault . . .

Client as Little One: I want to get away from here.

When asked by the therapist whether she could do that on her own, her answer is yes.

Therapist: Look for a place where you feel safe, where you can cry.
Client as Little One: I want to be accepted the way I am!

Finally, the dragon accompanies her into the woods where there are many animals. When invited by the therapist to establish a safe boundary all around, the four-year-old sets up an energy wall protecting her on all sides. Now she is safe. The therapist informs the Little One that from now on she can stay there, just being a child, growing up safely, and being cared for, so she can become big and strong.

The therapist also keeps speaking English with the four-year-old, who is laughing and is obviously happy when addressed in English. When the therapist says good-bye, the Little One says: Thank you . . . Bye-bye! (and she waves goodbye).

After this intervention, adult Chantal also feels freer, her legs feeling lighter.

Therapist: You are not alone, Chantal, you have the dragon. If you feel like it, you can pay the Little One a visit once in a while.

The client is very touched and weeps, telling the therapist that reconciliation has happened.

Therapist: Who knows, maybe the grownup will now also start learning or speaking English.

Here, the therapist was able to speak the four-year-old's language, but this is rather an exception and not a requirement. It is important to remember that the young ego state probably does not understand the language, or only part of it, and therefore needs a translator. In this case the therapist could not have asked the client whether she would translate because she had forgotten the English language. But she could have asked *what part* could translate for the Little One or could make sure that the four-year-old understood everything.

There are also ego states that do not speak for other reasons, for example, because they were not allowed to speak about the trauma back then. In such cases, they can be helped to establish their voice by asking a strong ego state for help, that is, connecting them with a part that is not subject to this "vow of silence" and can speak for them vicariously.

Dealing with Dissociation in Ego State Therapy

It has been mentioned several times that dissociation in people affected by trauma mostly represents a coping strategy learned in childhood. If the pain and/or the threat were overwhelming, the child took refuge in dissociation. Or, in Porges' perspective: Fight or flight were not possible, resulting in freeze response. If the freeze is not dissolved, these defense mechanisms are automatically reactivated in later stress situations.

When the client threatens to dissociate, this means that a part has emerged that wants to protect one or more anxious or suffering ego states.

Therapists can put a chair next to them, making this protecting part vicariously a co-therapist, and say:

"I can see that there is a very helpful part wanting to protect you." Then, turning to the chair: "Thank you for being there and looking out for the protection of X (the client). You have helped him since childhood and over and over and even now you are there instantly. I am also here to help. I would like you to stay, listen and, if necessary, help out. But now I would like to ask you to stay next to me and just listen. Afterwards I would be happy to find out more about you." Subsequently, the therapist addresses the part suffering or feeling overwhelmed by fear directly and empowers it, allowing for a corrective experience. If this was successful, the therapist can begin to negotiate new strategies with the Retro-State responsible for the dissociation, i.e., an ego state that is stuck or frozen in the past (Emmerson, 2014).

Often these protective parts are full of anger. Recognizing this anger as a defense strategy means appreciating the ego state's intention behind it and thus bringing it in. Moreover, we have the possibility to explore the anger via body sensations, resolving it and allowing it to transform into healthy self-assertion. How to deal with anger is described in a separate section in Chapter 5.

Utilizing Dissociation

Sometimes clients are too afraid to approach a traumatic experience. They fear being destabilized and overwhelmed by powerlessness and panic again. Here the therapist can use the dissociation and ask helping ego states to deal with the trauma contents instead of the client. Along the lines of Luise Reddemann (2007), an observing state ("inner observer") can also be invited to attend to the frightened or hurt ego states, while all suffering parts are safely on holiday or in a secure place. With strongly dissociative clients, Sandra Paulsen (2009) also suggests using an "amnesic barrier" to maintain the stability of the client. The everyday personality remains responsible for coping with everyday life and, via the amnesic barrier, is spared – dissociated from the traumatic contents – while other ego states deal with the pain or terror of the trauma until it is eased. In this way, dissociation or an amnesic barrier can be utilized so the everyday personality can keep its function.

Therapists do not need to know which procedure is exactly the right one. If they know various possibilities, they can suggest them to the clients or ask the inner team in the conference room for the right procedure.

The following case study illustrates how dissociation can be utilized in coping with trauma.

In our first session, 17-year-old Laura reports having a lot of stress and pressure at school because her performance was dropping drastically. She vomits once a week and is suffering from scary breathing problems (hyperventilation) that have been checked medically, with no organic reason identified.

Initially, coughing triggered the nausea, but now she puts her finger in her throat, feeling a relief from pressure and stress.

The symptoms originate in two traumatic experiences: Two years before, her mother's life was in jeopardy because of a life-threatening operation. At the same time, Laura had sex for the first time with her boyfriend, who was not very understanding. He wanted sex and she could not say no, so she let it happen, and her boyfriend left her afterwards, apologizing later. Lately she has had dreams about this ex-boyfriend apologizing.

Due to the high level of stress, the therapist decides to use trance. During this fantasy journey she keeps asking the client about her images, in order to be able to accompany her in as custom-fit a way as possible. This imagination emerges: The strains she is experiencing are heavy, hard stones that Laura packs in a backpack and deposits in a grey safe in a mountain cave, which she reaches after having hiked over a high plateau. After this trance she feels relieved.

In the second session she reports having felt good for a few days, but then experiencing her breathing problems again, suddenly not being able to breathe while learning.

The therapist shows her how she can calm and balance herself via *over-energy correction* (crossing her limbs). This is followed by another trance, which the therapist records on Laura's mobile, so she can listen to it at home. She communicates with Laura, or rather her unconscious, through ideomotor signals so as not to interrupt the flow of her words when she listens to it later. In this trance, a safe place is installed.

In the third session, Laura reports that she practiced the over-energy correction and was able to calm down immediately. After school, she listened to the recording of the safe place and fell asleep while listening. She had even used the exercise with the safe once in a while, and it had also worked well. Laura obviously has enough resources, and her self-regulation already works very well. Further, she has found an inner helper, the Teddybear, and established it as a resource. Now, the therapist explains to her that 15-year-old Laura must still be caught in the bad situation with the ex-boyfriend and that she should be rescued from this situation. She asks her whether she feels capable of doing so, maybe with the support of her inner helper, Teddybear? Laura says no.

Therapist: Could Teddybear do it instead of you?
              Laura nods.
Therapist: Does it need support or can it do it on its own?
Client: It can do it on its own.

Now the therapist accompanies Laura on the inner stage to her safe place where she is protected, left in peace, upon her request, and where she does not notice anything until the therapist contacts her again at a later state.

Then, the therapist speaks directly to the Teddybear (the client answers as Teddybear). Teddybear enters the situation where 15-year-old Laura is lying in bed with her ex-boyfriend. Teddybear saves her and brings her to a secret safe place: A tree house with a golden retriever, furnished nicely, and warm. Next to it is a swimming pool with cleansing healing water. (The swimming pool is Laura's idea; the cleansing healing and empowering water is suggested by the therapist, as well as the magical boundary around the tree house.) Moreover, the therapist suggests somebody who will accompany the 15-year-old from now on, supporting her with their wise advice and nourishing her, so that she can discover her sexuality at her own pace. A fairy appears who will take on these tasks from now on. Only when the corrective experience has been completed for the 15-year-old does the therapist say goodbye to her, Teddybear, and the fairy, and contacts Laura in her safe place again. The client is still feeling safe and secure there and obviously did not notice any of the "rescue mission."

In the fourth session, Laura reports that everything is easier for her. Further, she says that stress and pressure have decreased compared to before. She says, I wouldn't have considered it possible. Still, sometimes, the burden would come back, nearly making her cry. This means that the corrective experience has not yet been completed. The therapist remembers Laura's statement in the first session that she often dreamed of her ex-boyfriend apologizing. She asks Laura whether she still needs her ex-boyfriend to make amends on the inner stage and who could be the one to confront him. In a dialogue on the inner stage, her ex-boyfriend regrets and apologizes. Yet this is still not enough. Only when he receives an electronic tag, giving him an electric shock as soon as he thinks of hurting someone, does Laura feel safety in her chest and belly.

In the fifth and last session, Laura reports having felt very good since the last session, and not once having felt bad, not even in the evenings. Vomiting and shortage of breath have disappeared completely. She is cheerful again, has good life energy, and her school grades have improved.

Therapist: What has helped you most?
Client: Practicing over-energy correction and listening to the recorded trance.

This case study excerpt illustrates again how important self-regulation is, the ability to self-soothe. Since the client was obviously too afraid to be confronted with the traumatic scene directly, dissociation could be utilized. While Laura was protected and taken care of in a safe place, a helper ego state took over the rescue instead of her, here in the form of the teddy bear. Also, through this intervention, the danger of destabilization due to overwhelm was averted. Accordingly, the client had no memory of the corrective experience in the following session, yet she did notice the big difference now because her overall condition had improved.

Repairing Violated Boundaries

Our mostly unconscious awareness of boundaries (and this is true for any person) is shaped by the experiences during our development with the environment, involving all our senses such as seeing, hearing smelling, feeling, sense of balance, pain sensation, and self-awareness. Unpleasant or painful feedback tends to lead to withdrawal, positive feedback encourages one to explore the environment, thus expanding our own boundaries. Awareness of boundaries is constantly being newly shaped according to life experiences and the sensory messages we receive. The more positive and empowering these experiences are, the more stable one's own boundaries are experienced, and the more protected, safe, active, and self-effective individuals feel in their environment. This tangible boundary constitutes a nearly palpable, physiologically perceptible three-dimensional space (Scaer, 2001), resembling a bubble or sphere.

With every shock trauma, a violation of boundaries happens. What symptoms do people show whose boundaries have been violated? They feel exposed, defenseless, as if having no skin, reacting hyper-sensitively to sounds, light, or other stimuli. Stimulus satiation can alternate with rigidity. People with violated boundaries have a hard time setting boundaries with other people and also find it difficult to notice other people's boundaries.

Therefore, *repairing and strengthening boundaries* is another important element in trauma therapy, especially in the treatment of early childhood trauma and dissociation, where the violation of boundaries plays a central role. Clients learn to establish their personal boundaries, verbally, territorially – or physically and energetically. Gradually, they attain strong and healthy self-assertion, having started out with an inflexible or unclear, blurred perception of boundaries.

At the beginning of the therapy, even before knowing about any violation of boundaries (and also later during the treatment), therapists should check in with the clients as to the angle and distance they should sit from them. The therapist wants to show respect and be cognizant of the space in which clients feel safe. Levine (2017) suggests having clients sit at a 45-degree angle from the therapist. Thus, they can decide themselves, whether and for how long they want to keep eye contact with the therapist. Moreover, both are looking in the same direction.

In the final chapter you can find practical instructions and exercises for repairing boundaries.

Boundaries that have not been repaired can also be the reason why hurt younger parts cannot be soothed and integrated completely. This is illustrated by the continuation of the case study with the 40-year-old client with nine-year-old ego state Vera from Chapter 2.

In the seventh session, the client wants to take care of Vera. First, Vera needs more safety. The grandfather is still too close in the cage she had given him during an earlier session. She sends him to another planet, from where he can not return, where he has to work and build for others. But it still does not feel completely good. Therapist: What else is there? The therapist encourages the client to simply notice what she senses in her body, such as, for instance, impulses for micro-movements. There are small impulses of pushing away with the hands, which the therapist supports verbally, slowing them down: Let your hands do what they want to do but very slowly, even slower, in slow motion. Very good! Yes exactly.

A long process of pushing away with both hands ensues, during which the client's breath keeps stalling. Very good! Continue breathing! Exactly! Breathe. The client uses her fists to hit in slow motion, her hands pushing away. And her feet and legs defend themselves with slow but powerful kicks, accompanied by the client's weeping. The therapist keeps inviting her to pause and feel: What is it like now? She responds, Grandfather is lying on the floor. I want to spit at him! The therapist supports this as well. The client makes gestures of spitting. The slow movements of her extremities become more fluent and harmonious, seeming like a liberation dance that her body is performing on her seat. Then she spontaneously expresses sentences like: I am strong! It is liberating! The therapist notes these on a piece of paper as well, which she hands to the client at the end of the session. The grandfather now has to go to a labor camp with fences.

Then: This is good, but I still don't feel quite safe. The mother could break down. I have to take care of her. Therapist: What does the mother need? After exploring and pondering carefully, the client concludes the following: The mother needs a nursing sanatorium, where she is taken care of and is safe. Now it is okay! The brother also needs to be cared for in order to be safe, in his own tree house. Only now can Vera enjoy her cabin, noticing her environment properly and seeing what is there. It is super beautiful, she says, quite thrilled. The client reports at the end of the session: The final image is beautiful and sensual. The body process touched me deeply. Finally, I'm able to defend myself!

The therapist is curious to hear her feedback at the beginning of the next session: The last session was great, I'm extremely grateful. The experience of self-defense was important. I'm allowed to defend myself. That set a lot in motion and gave me strength! It's interesting, when done in slow motion, the individual sequences of experience become clearer, for example disgust or distaste, but also strength and muscle tension. Through the slow movements one feels oneself much more!

The client also reports about the effects in her everyday life: There's a lot more joy and vitality, liveliness, courage. She pasted slips of paper with the sentences, "I am strong!" and "I'm okay just the way I am" to her mirror and kept looking at them over and over. In the meantime, she "visited" Vera, reporting, "It's nice that she is doing well!"

The client describes vividly how, by slowing down the movements, all the different feelings such as fear and disgust are decoupled from the defense strategies blocked in the body, thus allowing for healthy self-assertion.

At the beginning, as well as later during therapy, it is always helpful with clients having experienced violation of boundaries to create boundaries three dimensionally in space and physically, by having them show their boundaries with a rope or chalk. These are then checked for their correctness – Are the distances right? Has the client taken enough space?

In Chapter 8, readers will find exact instructions as well as a case study of how boundaries can be newly established and thus experienced physically in the section "Repairing boundaries."

The following description of a live demonstration during an advanced training illustrates how to proceed with establishing boundaries.

Fifty-year-old Olaf has laid out his personal boundaries, having been invited by the therapist to do so. With the help of the therapist, he explores them from the direction he considers to be safe and changes and forms them according to his feeling. When the therapist begins walking slowly along the circle of his boundaries in different directions and moves to the left side of the client, he freezes. His posture stiffens as if he were in danger. He himself is surprised about this arousal. The therapist moves back again to the safe zone, inviting Olaf to notice and describe his sensations. Suddenly, memories of a high-speed fall from his bicycle surface. The front tire had exploded and Olaf had been incredibly lucky when he fell on his left side and was only slightly injured. While he is talking, the therapist invites him to also explore his sensations. Then she carefully moves back to the left side, pausing and allowing Olaf to feel his sensations, and then moves back into the safe zone. She keeps going back and forth until the left side also feels safe and protected to Olaf and the new boundary is established.

Trauma and Dissociation through Rejection and Neglect

Dissociative phenomena are not always triggered by shock trauma. Prolonged emotional and physical neglect can also be the reason. In his lecture at the European congress of hypnosis in Manchester (2017), Camillo Loriedo, Professor of psychiatry at the University of Rome and president of the Italian Society for Hypnosis, pointed out that neglect in the first few years can lead to dissociation.

A child needs bonding to survive. This attachment can become a problem, if the parents show *unpredictable* behavior, such as violence, over-stimulation, scaring the child, superiority, weakness, confusion, dependency, neglect, seduction, abandonment, overstepping boundaries, callousness, debasement, accusation, humiliation, absence, psychosis, sexual perversion, sadism, overcontrol, or impulsiveness. Some parents, who meet such criteria show clinical dissociative disorders reinforcing the unpredictability that the child has to suffer. In long-term studies, children with parents with a disorganized attachment style showed significantly more dissociative symptoms later in life (Dalenberg et al., 2012). The parents of these children are usually severely traumatized themselves, for instance by war, violence or neglect, and, through their insecure and avoiding attachment behavior, are responsible for gross emotional neglect of their children although they may try hard, want the best for their children, and mean well.

What Forms of Neglect are there?

In many clients, signs of emotional neglect will appear during the therapeutic process, and, in severe cases, also the neglect of physical needs. Very often you will find a lack of presence of the attachment figures, which can be associated with moral neglect and a lack of protection.

Ogawa et al. (1997) have described the consequences of parents not being psychologically accessible for their children. Their study showed that neglect in the first two years of a child's life leads to clinically relevant dissociative symptoms. Other studies also illustrate the after-effects of neglect in childhood. If, in severe cases, no caring object can be internalized, due to a lack of attention and care by the primary attachment figure, the child's organism resorts to auto-sensual satisfaction (*autistic contiguous position*), whereby a mental space is fabricated that can exist independently of the presence of other people (Ogden, 1989). The associated rhythmic and self-comforting ways of behavior for self-soothing are also expressed in later behavioral addictions.

A dysfunctional family pattern with neglect can lead to somatoform disorders such as bulimia nervosa and to borderline disorders as an adolescent or adult. The study by Mehta et al. (2009) with adopted adolescents having been neglected severely during early childhood and a non-adopted, non-neglected control group showed that both the volume of the grey and the white matter of the brain was significantly smaller in the neglected individuals. This finding offers further proof of how important safe attachment behavior of the parents – and oxytocin – is for the development of the child's brain.

In families where there is neglect, a lot can be gained by drawing the family's interest to the individual so that they can be seen and accepted by the other family members, showing the family system what it had lost for a long time and how valuable it can be to re-include the neglected family member (Loriedo, 2017).

What if the family is not available? Fortunately, with Ego State therapy, there is the possibility of creating the conditions for such "rehabilitation" to happen on the inner stage, by supporting and generating safe attachments intra-psychically, thus allowing for a corrective experience and development.

Emmerson calls the emotional state of the rejected neglected child "vaded with rejection" (2014). The child, overwhelmed by rejection, is flooded with the feeling of not being good enough. It feels unloved, constantly judged or condemned by others, anxious about what others might think, or has the feeling of only being lovable when performing. This personality part is always demanding validation by others or compares itself with others, trying to be "better." This search for acknowledgment and validation can compromise or prevent social contacts, making for excessive competitiveness and leading to massive self-doubts. Behind this lies a deep longing to be loved unconditionally.

In Ego State therapy, it is irrelevant how the relationship parent-child was objectively lived. The child "vaded with rejection" felt incapable of experiencing an unconditionally accepting relationship with one or both parents. However, this does not mean that the parents did not provide it, it only means that the child did not experience it as unconditional love. The experiences and attempts of the client to resolve the problem are what is relevant for therapy. The client is always right, as Maggie Phillips liked to say.

Another dysfunctional coping strategy besides those just mentioned is anorexia nervosa. With this clinical picture, parents frequently tend to be over-protective, pampering the child and supporting it. Often there is also a rejected ego state in one of the parents. They want their child to be really well. The child must become a perfect child, anything else is not acceptable. In the parents' endeavor, they unconsciously put the focus on achievement, and so the child misses out on experiencing loving accepting care. The child desperately seeks emotional connection and unconditional acceptance, and supposedly achieves that by no longer eating. This triggers unfavorable dynamics that are now difficult to interrupt. In an attempt to make the child safe and healthy again, the parents exert pressure, force the child to eat, which only reinforces her refusal, unconsciously fueled by the need for unconditional connection. Thus, unintentionally, they prevent therapy from progressing. With anorexia nervosa, it is therefore important to also work with the parents on the outer stage, not only with the rejecting introjects inside. The therapist can encourage the parents to put the focus on vulnerability and a loving relationship with each other, and more on acceptance of the whole personality than on achievement. This also includes ego state work with the rejected part of the parents. Only when they feel safe and "good enough" can they become unconditionally loving parents. The inner acceptance of the parents helps children to accept themselves as they are.

With bulimia (without anorexia) the focus is somewhat different: A rejected ego state wears itself out by competing with others, to quench their longing for accepting love. The driving force behind bulimia is also the need to be superior to others – inferiority triggers fear. The figure of another person, perceived as being "more beautiful," sparks the strong desire to lose weight. Normally, clients with bulimia quickly respond to the release and rehabilitation of the rejected ego state and can change their behavior relatively quickly – as opposed to the persistent patterns and systemic factors with anorexia nervosa.

With both clinical pictures, you have to also work with the state causing the unwanted behavior (starving with anorexia, or gorging and vomiting with bulimia), after having integrated the rejected personality part. Emmerson calls this part the "Retro Avoiding State," meaning a state that is stuck in the past and is trying to avoid painful feelings. This part developed in the past to avoid the bad feelings of being rejected.

Rehabilitation: From Rejection to Unconditional Love

The states overwhelmed by rejection perpetuate the negative experience of being unworthy, incapable, or not lovable. According to Emmerson (2014), the impression of a rejecting introject continues to exist. This is why a state overwhelmed by rejection, feeling unloved or not appreciated, needs to experience that every child deserves unconditional love and that it is not the child's fault if that love was not offered or received. In doing so, the *feeling* of not being good enough must be touched instead of just thinking about it. If the client stays on the intellectual level, the state cannot come into consciousness. Therefore, the therapist doesn't ever request: Go back to the first time you felt like this! This type of instruction results in the client having to think, taking them out of the *felt experience* and making them take distance from this state. Rather, the therapist asks for a very *specific situation*, an exact moment when the state was experienced. An answer such as, Whenever I'm sitting in my kitchen, is not enough. Once a specific situation in which the client experiences this unwanted feeling or the behavior aiming at avoiding this feeling in everyday life is brought forward, by "bridging" – meaning the exploration of the body sensations and feelings associated with the state experiencing rejection – the therapist should speak to this state directly and encourage it to express completely and to name its feelings. This state experiencing rejection now tells the rejecting introject, for which an empty chair can be set up, in direct speech everything that is on its mind. According to Emmerson, when an ego state is overwhelmed by rejection, the dialogue with the introject should always be guided. The therapist might say: "He is not really here, so now you have the opportunity to tell him anything you like!" If self-expression is possible within the safe space, *empowerment* happens, so that the rejected state is released from the extremely shameful and powerless position of being outcast. Then, the therapist asks the client to sit on the chair of the introject, addressing the introject directly:

"Mother, what do you want to answer your son?" The client then speaks as the mother, saying for example: "I shouldn't ever have given birth to you." Or: "I was so lonely and was so afraid of doing everything wrong." In response, the therapist does not try to change the introject's mind, since this would only lead to a power struggle between therapist and introject. Rather, the therapist asks the client to return to their seat, addressing the client again as the rejected ego state. Oh dear, I understand why you felt like that. Your mother was in no way capable of giving you unconditional love. However, every child deserves to be loved, no matter whether they are good or make mistakes. You also have the right to receive the love that you deserve just as any child does. This acknowledgment changes the feeling of the rejected state. I am not lovable, becomes, my mother was not able to give me the love I deserved. This is a deep shift. If the state has experienced this shift, another empowering step follows: Therapists let the clients decide whether they still want the introject, i.e., the mother, in their inner space or not. The inner space does not refer to the whole inner stage, as with Emmerson's Resource therapy, but rather the inner space of the ego state on the inner stage that it can shape and contain according to its own wishes through the corrective experience. No matter what the state decides, having the possibility *to decide*, provides greater power. Normally, states no longer want the introject with them in their inner space.

The following dialogue between the child ego state, Sandra, and the mother introject illustrates these steps, but without using chairs (see Chapter 5).

Therapist:	What would you like to tell your mother, Sandra? You can now finally express yourself and say anything you like. Tell your mother directly!
Client as Sandra (to the mother):	It makes me really angry that you act as though everything were okay, when it's not true! It makes me so angry that you don't really live! (The client's father died when she was seven years old. Her childhood and youth were clouded by her mother's grief.)
Therapist to mother:	What do you answer your daughter?
Client (as mother):	I'm trying hard to make everything normal. I'm afraid that it will all get worse, that you, Sandra, might fall ill or take drugs or that something bad might happen!
Therapist to Sandra:	What's that like for you?
Client as Sandra:	I feel like I'm not normal, not okay the way I am.
Therapist to mother:	What do you reply to that?
Client (as mother):	I'm sorry, I don't want that. You're okay.
Therapist:	Tell your daughter again that she is okay the way she is!

The mother repeats it.

Therapist:	What is that like for you now, Sandra?
Client as Sandra:	That is good for me. I'm healthy. It's nice and at the same time it hurts.
Therapist:	It hurts that the fear of mother has become your own fear, that you had to have that fear for so long. But, fortunately, that is over for good now. You are wonderful just the way you are, whether you are angry, sad, or cheerful. You have the right to have all these feelings and to also express them. Do you understand, Sandra, that it is over? That from now on you can be angry and that it is okay for your mother?

Client as Sandra:	It is a tentative understanding. I still need something from mama.
Therapist:	What do you need?
Client as Sandra:	That she holds me at my shoulders and tells me she's sorry.
Therapist to Mother:	Are you willing to do that? The mother confirms. Then go to your daughter, hold her at her shoulders and tell her: I'm sorry. You are wonderful just the way you are. I love you even when you are angry!
Client (as Mother):	I'm sorry. You are wonderful the way you are. I love you very much. You can be angry.
Therapist:	What is that like for you, Sandra?
Client as Sandra:	It's empowering. I've calmed down. I am a bit tired. It was so stressful with this fear.

When asked by the therapist what she still needs, Sandra says she would like to be in the meadow with Mother and all the relatives without fear and anger. She says: We are both tired and sad, but it's okay.

The therapist now addresses the adult client:

Therapist:	Does Sandra now have everything she needs?
Client:	She's still doubtful when she hears her mother tell her she loves her very much.
Therapist:	Could you tell or give Sandra something more so she can become safer?
Client (to Sandra):	I also love you, take your time, nothing bad is going to happen. You can just try out . . . being angry.
Therapist:	I'm glad that Sandra is finally in good hands with her relatives and that Mother and you are telling her that she is okay, that you and all the others love her.

Then the therapist asks the client to, in her mind, go back to the initial situation. She feels a pleasant warmth. She describes comfortable warmth: I'm standing straight, feeling more safe and bigger! It feels good, normal.

Parentified clients having had to take care of their parents in childhood often develop a bad conscience regarding the introject, i.e., worry about it when they have sent it out of their inner space. The therapist can then suggest a place outside where it is in good hands and can stay for good, as illustrated in the case study with the ego state "Vera," wherein she has her cozy cabin, and Mother was placed in a sanitarium and her brother is given his tree house. Only there, the formerly rejected and overwhelmed ego state could really be integrated and find peace, when the mother and the brother introject were taken care of. Now is the right moment to bring in one or more helping supporting states, if wanted. The decision lies with the client, who intuitively knows what is useful. The therapist asks the client what the formerly rejected state still needs and who could possibly support it. The helping state is then asked to hug the rejected one, and the rejected one can be invited to also hug the helper and to feel what that is like. Now the empowered, formerly rejected state can get a new name, if the old one (i.e., Unloved) no longer fits. Maybe the state now wants to be called "In Good Hands" and thus from then on, the therapist calls it by that name. The intervention is only completed once the client feels distinctly better in the specific situation explored at the beginning leading to the rejected state. Emmerson (2014) calls the checking of the specifically imagined problematic situation at the end the "Imagery Check."

After having integrated the ego state overwhelmed by rejection, the therapist continues by negotiating with the part responsible for the unwanted behavior stuck in the past (Retro Avoiding). This is about creating an alliance, similar to the work with the destructively acting ego state, to increase its readiness for change. The understating becomes that the formerly rejected part has been rehabilitated, that it is still wanted with its intention to help and that it will be appreciated by the other ego states and by the client when it changes its behavior. Thus, this once-rejected part will be ready to cooperate and join the inner team, and it will be welcomed.

Instructions for the work with *rejected and avoiding* ego states as well as with the *Retro* States[2] triggering the unwanted behavior along the lines of Emmerson (2015) can be found in Chapter 8.

Notes

1 This therapy session was held in French.
2 Retro states are considered the villains in the intrapsychic system because they use inappropriate or even harmful behavior in order to achieve goals (*retro original*) or in order to protect consciousness from being overwhelmed by undesirable emotional states through avoidance (*retro avoiding*).

References

Dalenberg, C. J., D. H. Gleaves, M. J. Dorahy, E. Cardena, E. B. Carlson, B. L. Brand, R. J. Loewenstein, P. A. Frewen, & D. Spiegel (2012): Evaluation of the Evidence for the Trauma and Fantasy Models of Dissociation. *Psychological Bulletin, 138(3)*: 550–588.
Emmerson, G. (2015): *Learn Resource therapy. Clinical Qualification Student Training Manual.* Victoria: Old Golden Point.
Emmerson, G. (2014): *Resource Therapy. The Complete Guide with Case Examples & Transcripts.* Victoria: Old Golden Point.
Kain, K. & Terrell, S. (2018): *Nurturing Resilience. Helping Clients Move Forward from Developmental Trauma. An Alternative Somatic Approach.* North Atlantic Books.
Levine, P. (2017): Shame and Pride, Seminar in Weggis, Switzerland (12–15 August 2017).
Levine, P. (2015): *Trauma and Memory: Brain and Body in a Search for the Living Past: A Practical Guide for Understanding and Working with Traumatic Memory.* North Atlantic Books U.S.

Levine, P. (2010): *In an Unspoken Voice: How the Body Releases Trauma and Restores Goodness*. Berkeley: North Atlantic Books.

Levine, P. (1997): *Waking the Tiger – Healing Trauma*. Berkeley: North Atlantic Books.

Loriedo, C. (2017): *Using Hypnosis with Families*. (Keynote, 19th Congress European Society of Hypnosis, Manchester, 23–26 August 2017).

Mehta, M. A., Golembo, N. I., Nosarti, C., Colvett. E., Mota, A., Williams, S. C. R., Rutter, M., & Sonuga-Barke, E. J. S. (2009): Amygdala, Hippocampal and Corpus Callosum Size Following Severe Early Institutional Deprivation: The English and Romanian Adoptees Study Pilot. *Journal of Child Psychology and Psychiatry, 50(8)*: 943–951.

Ogawa, J. R., Sroufe, L. A., Weinfield, N. S., Carlson, E. A., & Egeland, B. (1997): *Development and the Fragmented Self: Longitudinal Study of Dissociative Symptomatology in a Nonclinical Sample*. Development and Psychopathology, *9*: 855–879.

Ogden, T. H. (1989): On the Concept of an Autistic-contiguous Position. *The International Journal of Psycho-Analysis, 70*: 127–140.

Paulsen, S. (2009): *Looking through the Eyes of Trauma and Dissociation. An Illustrated Guide for EMDR Therapists and Clients*. BookSurge Publishing.

Phillips, M. (2016): *How to Heal Trauma and Pain Through the Body: Somatic Psychotherapy Level 3*, (Seminar in Zurich, 30 September–1 October 2016).

Phillips, M. & Frederick, C. (1995): *Healing the Divided Self. Clinical and Ericksonian Hypnotherapy: Clinical and Ericksonian Hypnotherapy for Dissociative Conditions*. W.W. Norton & Company, Inc.

Reddemann, L. (2007): *Imagination als heilsame Kraft. Zur Behandlung von Traumafolgen mit ressourcenorientierten Verfahren*. Stuttgart: Klett-Cotta.

Scaer, R. (2001). *The Body Bears the Burden: Trauma, Dissociation and Disease*. Routledge.

Schmidt, G. (2010): *Liebesaffären zwischen Problem und Lösung. Hypnosystemisches Arbeiten in schwierigen Kontexten*. Heidelberg: Carl Auer.

van der Kolk, B. (2017). *How Trauma Lodges in the Body*. (Interview On Being: www.onbeing.org).

Chapter 5

The Energy of Anger

Utilizing the Energy of Anger

Aggression and anger are emotions that are part of basic defense mechanisms, and they serve self-assertion. It is important to acknowledge this function of asserting oneself and setting a boundary. With clients who were not able to defend themselves successfully in the past, therapists should welcome aggression and anger in the therapeutic process. Therapists can reframe anger as an important power and resource and utilize the strong energy associated with it and transform it into healthy self-assertion. Clients are often surprised about this reframing of anger. There are also clients who consider fits of rage, which are judged negatively by their environment, as strength because they give them power. It is the strategy of defense with which they have learned to assert themselves. Therapeutic steps with this retro state are only possible if clients reject that behavior and want to change it (Emmerson, 2014).

Inappropriate Anger

If anger is expressed in undesirable behavior like uncontrolled fits of rage, Emmerson (2014) suggests first acknowledging the good intention of this state of anger (retro state) and then looking for a "resource state" that can defend itself in an appropriate way, which is not always easy to find. If, for example, a state is needed that can assert itself or help the client to set boundaries more easily, without being blinded by rage, the therapist might ask the client to describe what it would be like to assert oneself. Or, the therapist might invite the client to imagine a person who is good at setting boundaries and to describe this person in all detail.

Once a vivid description is given, the therapist says: Wait a minute! What may I call you, you who are talking about self-assertion and knows so much about it? Would you help X (the client) to self-assert in such a way that there are no negative consequences for them? Then the therapist suggests

DOI: 10.4324/9781003460602-6

to the state of rage (the retro state) an alternative or new role. At this point, the therapist does not ask the state whether it wants to take on the new role, rather, a seed is planted for this idea, with questions such as: What do you suppose X (the client) and the other ego states might think of you if you were to apply this new strategy?

Retro states are convinced they can only use this one strategy and that the other parts and the client will never like or appreciate them, yet it is amazing how quickly their attitude changes when they find out that there is a chance of them being liked and appreciated, first by the therapist and then by other states and the client. This effect is reinforced when the other parts tell the retro state directly that they will like it with its new role. (The instructions for working with retro states can be found in Chapter 8.)

The following therapy section demonstrates the transformation of a retro state from an opponent to a team player, and also illustrates the variety of ways, sometimes even in rather strange figures, inner parts can present themselves. The therapist explores and focuses on the reactions of the different states and of the client, on the resolution of the inner conflict and, as a result, the healing experience of integration.

The 48-year-old female client reports how fear and resignation determine her life: I'm afraid a tumor is growing inside of me, and then everything hurts, and nothing else exists except this fear! It is stronger than me! I'm walking on thin ice, without roots, no confidence, losing my connection to life. . . .

Therapist:	Where do you feel that?
Client:	On my skin, a tingling, I'm nervous, my breathing is shallow, I'm like a deer that is frightened.
Therapist:	How old do you feel?
Client:	Small, but I am not a human being, I am like a Will-o'-the-wisp.
Therapist:	May I speak to this Will-o'-the-wisp? The client agrees.
Therapist:	May I call you Will-o'-the-wisp? Yes? Will-o'-the-wisp, you are frightened, aren't you?
Client as Will-o'-the-wisp:	I am flickering about like a little ghost.
Therapist:	What do you need?
Client:	A space where I am safe.

The therapist explains to the Will-o'-the-wisp that it is safe and can change its environment in such a way that it feels safe.

Client as *Will-o'-* *the-wisp:*	What I want is peace and quiet, a haven to land . . . There is food, green soil, sound resonating, a boundary, trees at the edge . . . it is a haven.
Therapist:	Will-o'-the-wisp, I'm sorry that you had to wander about. Like all parts, you deserve to be safe and to feel good and rooted. Then addressing the client: What is it like now?
Client:	It takes time, but it is much better . . . But there is something in the back, struggling. The center . . . the bridge is closed . . . interfering with breathing . . . I'm getting a headache . . .
Therapist:	Two parts are wanting to talk. Which parts are they?
Client:	One is my head, the other something rising . . .
Therapist:	Whose turn is it first? The client mentions, "Rising." The therapist asks Rising directly what it needs.
Rising:	I need free passage. I know where I want to go.

To this, the head replies: That's too fast, you are passing me over . . . Stop! I have to protect; I am the Border Guard!

Therapist:	Border Guard, I'm glad you're here. You seem to be an important protection.
Border *Guard:*	I'm grumpy and rather fed up with always having to lower the barrier. I also have other qualities. I'm frustrated, I'm looking for another job and, after all this time, I want to be appreciated.
Therapist:	Rising, would you like Border Guard if he were no longer hindering but only protecting?

To begin with, Rising cannot imagine that. After a while she approves.

Therapist:	Tell Border Guard directly!
Rising to *Border* *Guard:*	It would be great if you could open the barrier and accompany me up, show me the way, open the space and set the pace, that would be helpful.
Therapist:	Rising, would you like Border Guard if he did that?
Rising:	I cannot imagine that yet, I'm finding it difficult to say something . . .
Therapist:	And you, Border Guard?
Border *Guard:*	I would like connection, that would be much more exciting than just standing here and always hindering. The therapist asks Border Guard to tell Rising directly.

Border Guard to Rising:	I would like to accompany you and, together, achieve something bigger, we can only do that together.
Rising:	Oh, I'm so glad. It would be great, Border Guard, if we were a team: Protection instead of hindrance.
Therapist:	You have all the time you need . . .
Client weeps:	Cooperation is beginning . . .

The therapist accompanies this process of integration with the following words: Your body can let cooperation and connection happen now . . . allowing for anything that's stagnating to flow again and yet being protected.

Client:	It is nice, they're flowing and engaging together . . .
Therapist:	Will-o'-the-wisp, where are you? How are you doing?
Will-o'-the-wisp:	I'm more . . . calm.
Therapist:	Will-o'-the-wisp, are you also with the others?
Will-o'-the-wisp:	I'm shifting my shape with the connection that is happening now.
Therapist:	Does the name Will-o'-the-wisp still fit? . . . No? What may I call you?
Will-o'-the-wisp:	My name is Ray of Light.
Therapist:	A nice name. Ray of Light, you can join Rising and Border Guard.
Ray of Light:	That's nice. Now I feel at home here. Before, I was always ejected.
Therapist:	It's not your fault, that you kept being thrown out. That probably had to do with the conflict between Border Guard and Rising . . .
Ray of Light:	I see myself as the center of this channel . . . It's nice, it is happening . . .
Therapist:	Take your time.
Ray of Light:	I know I belong here, but sometimes I forget.
Therapist:	You used to forget sometimes, but that's over now!

When two conflicting ego states want to be out at the same time, clients often get a headache, as seen in this example. This headache disappears just as spontaneously as it appears as soon as the inner conflict is resolved.

Angry Ego States

There are also angry ego states that have forgotten that they developed as a protection, for example, those identifying with the aggressor. They feel so strongly rejected by the client and the other ego states that they think they are in another body, so they keep taking their anger out on a weak and vulnerable ego state. Just like the perpetrator in the past, they feel overpowering and despise the weakness of the small "victim" states, torturing and blaming them (Paulsen, 2009). These, in turn, believe them, allowing them to intimidate them, as in the case study with the 62-year-old man in Chapter 4, in which "Scapegoat" suffered from experiencing the malicious "voices." In this case communicating with all ego states involved and with the client is essential. They must be informed that these inner dynamics belong to the past and are dysfunctional, and that they have the possibility to take on new roles and to be liked by the others. If therapists understand the original intention of the angry ego states, they can face them with openness and respect.

From Helplessness to Power

Ego State therapy offers many possibilities for corrective experiences with anger. Helen Watkins (1980) suggested *Silent Abreaction*, a very useful technique for hopeless situations or those that cannot be changed or where the client feels powerless. In these cases, silent abreaction can be liberating because the anger is acted out in a trance, in an imaginary way, and something can be done and changed. When using this technique, the therapist helps the client imagine the hopeless situation or the object of the anger as a figure or shape – for example, a huge rock blocking the way. Then clients try smashing the rock as hard as possible, with an appropriate imaginary instrument, until they feel it is enough. The abreaction is "silent" because the client does not scream and shout or flail about, but only imagines the scenario with intensity, doing the action in a trance, but staying quiet, which, neuro-physiologically, stimulates the same sensory and motor circuits as if acting. This technique can be adapted individually to the inner scenarios surfacing, accompanied by the therapist as a catharsis. It is very effective because, on the inner stage, a new corrective experience happens.

Empowerment through Expression

The following case study excerpt illustrates how expressing anger can empower and strengthen all ego states having experienced helplessness. Again, you can see how effective a combination of Ego State therapy and body therapies can be in healing trauma.

Twenty-one-year-old Marina had already been in therapy as a teenager because of problems with her parents. Thus, trust and a safe therapeutic relationship have already been installed.

In her first session she reports that after having had her first sexual experiences with her boyfriend, she had an indistinct feeling of having been sexually abused by her coach as a six-year-old child. She vaguely remembers being asked by her mother whether her coach had acted in a strange way towards her. At the time, Marina denied anything out of shame, she did not want her mother to notice anything. In fact, she remembers a scene in the dressing room where the coach stripped in front of her, but then her memory fades. Later she had been given a reward by her coach, because she was so good at rope skipping.

The therapist first informs Marina about trauma and memory, the involuntary psychophysiological mechanisms of the psyche and organism (psychoeducation), and then focusses on strengthening her resources. She asks, when, in daily life, does Marina feel the way she would like to feel more or less all the time? Marina replies, when she is with friends and can be a good friend to them. She feels that in her heart area and in her belly as a warm and pleasant feeling of happiness (*experience free of conflict*). Now Marina is asked to take the position of a dissociated observer where she can observe from a distance in which she feels safe (*inner observer*).

Therapist: Who can take care of the 6-year-old? Could you do that, Marina, from your position as an observer?

Marina shakes her head.

Therapist: Who could do that?
Client: An angel or a good girlfriend of mine.

While Marina remains in her role as an observer, the therapist tells six-year-old Marina that this is not happening now and that now she can actually get away. She wants to go to her nursery, the angel and her good friend accompanying her. She is given a cuddly toy, a bed with a warm blanket and a protective bubble as a safe boundary. The therapist suggests cleansing herself in order to heal, so the angel and the good friend help the six-year-old to take a shower (*corrective experience*).

After this intervention, Marina feels very "flabby" despite the dissociation using the position of an observer. The therapist invites her to take her time, after which she slowly starts feeling her legs again. The therapist supports her coming back into her body by asking Marina to gently press the balls of her feet on the ground when inhaling and letting go when exhaling (*grounding breathing exercise*).

Therapist:`   It is important that you take it easy after the session and in the next few days, and that you take your time and be careful with yourself. You have gone through very deep inner experiences needing time to heal. See yourself as a convalescent and take good care of yourself. Please send me an email in a few days and let me know how you are doing.

In her email, Marina writes: I took good care of myself, a great deal of sadness and anger have been coming up, mood swings, ups and downs. However, she does not feel it is necessary to make an additional appointment.

In the second session we focus on Marina's sadness and anger. Intense feelings of hatred towards the coach keep overwhelming her. She weeps. After strengthening her resources in a safe place, the therapist asks how the six-year-old is doing and is told that she is in the nursery playing, yet not feeling completely safe. When asked what she needs, Marina answers: A family, Daddy and Mummy, a brother . . . She is very sad, and also needs a grandma comforting her.

Only now is the six-year-old safe and hence the *corrective experience* complete, the fear overcome and uncoupled. Grownup Marina now feels strong, especially in her legs. Yet there is still a great deal of anger threatening to overwhelm her. The therapist invites Marina to hold the wrist of the therapist and press all her anger into it. Therapist: Don't worry, you can press as hard as you need to, I will say, "Stop," if it hurts. Together with the therapist, Marina takes a deep breath and presses her anger into the therapist's wrist when exhaling, being instructed by her to pause and rest, to sense what it feels like and whether another "round" is necessary. This *release* of anger is accompanied by intense sobbing. The therapist supports this process by reassuring her: Well done, that's it, now finally the anger can dissolve.

After this intervention Marina feels relieved, free, airy, especially in her feet. She notices a "congestion of the energy" in her head and chest. The therapist invites Marina to imagine inhaling through her feet and legs and exhaling through her chest and the top of her head and to try this a few times. After a few breathing cycles, her head and chest also feel light and pleasant. To complete the session, Marina goes to her safe place.

A few days later, Marina writes in an email: Thursday's session was incredibly good for me. Since then, I have been feeling very strong. That is a really, really nice feeling! Now I notice that the six-year-old is doing really well. It is good to know that and also feels really good. I am enjoying these positive feelings very much, using them to stock up my energy.

Releasing Anger from the Body

Somatic Experiencing® therapy offers the possibility of releasing pent-up anger in a controlled way, titrating the micromovements by slowly completing the blocked or inhibited defense strategy.

A good example is the case of the 40-year-old woman in Chapter 2 (and continued in Chapter 4) mauling and kicking the abusive grandfather, and also spitting at him.

The therapist even supports actions that are ethically not allowed and would be condemned by society if done for real, such as spitting, insulting, beating, kicking, hurting or even destroying, so the powerlessness and helplessness can be transformed into activity and the client may feel and experience self-efficacy. With sufferers who were not or are not able to defend themselves in real life or whose anger is directed *inwardly*, anything that helps the resolution of the traumatic experience should be allowed on the inner stage, in contrast to violent sufferers, because these actions on the inner stage are about self-defense, about completing protection and defense strategies that could not happen or got stuck. This must go on until the client feels good or feels that it is enough. With these imagined acts and the movements in slow motion, clients start sensing their strength and power, experiencing competence and control, and are able to step out of their victimhood, then spontaneously expressing sentences like: I can defend myself! I'm strong!

After the phase of self-assertion and marking one's boundaries, clients might be asked whether they still want the person (the object of their anger) in their inner space or in their inner environment. Usually, clients answer that they do not want them there unless something needs to be "finished," as in the example with the state "Sandra," which appears later in this chapter. Then the therapist can invite the client to inhale deeply and banish the unwanted person from their inner environment while exhaling. Clients often accompany this with noises or gestures. Only when the inner environment is completely safe does the therapist help the client to complete this inner experience.

Letting Anger Flow

If the anger is trapped as high excess energy in the body, the therapist can ask the client to hold the wrist of the therapist, the back of the chair, or a hard rubber ball (or another suitable object) and to let the anger pour into it, or to press hard into the object with every exhale, while reassuring them.

Like Peter Levine (2017), the author also uses so-called "Vibroswing Smovie Rings" to channel anger or to move out of freezing. Clients are asked to project all their anger into the rings, and then the therapist begins swinging the rings, together with the client, exhaling with noise. The movements of the client tend to be rather tentative at first but become more and more vigorous and powerful, and soon the shoulder and neck area start relaxing visibly. By allowing the client to occasionally rest and "sense" into it, titration happens, thus releasing the huge energy of anger carefully and yet with verve.

Anger may also be pressed and discharged into the armrests of a chair while exhaling, pausing and tracking sensations in between cycles of energy release, as described above. Another possibility for the therapist is to offer his or her wrist or a squeeze ball instead of the armrests.

Setting Boundaries – Letting Go

A client in his mid-40s is angry about "grousers" in his sports association, not doing anything but spreading untruths about him as the president. When the therapist asks him to notice his being angry and to stay with it, he becomes agitated, and finds it more difficult to breathe.

Therapist: What are your body sensations?
Client: There is a heaviness in my belly, like a big, rectangular stone.
Therapist: How big? Could you show me?

The client uses his hands to show a rectangle of about 20 × 40 cm.

Therapist: Stay with it for a moment and keep observing.
Client: It is bloated, an organic lump. There is congestion at the navel, as though it were tied together with a string. Below there is a huge bulge.

The therapist watches and waits.

Client: I'm very cross. I'd like to enjoy these summer days instead of getting so upset that I fall ill!
Therapist: Exactly. You were so much looking forward to these days and now there's this lump!
Client: In this lump there is also mucus, he continues, and that doesn't belong to me. The mucus has nothing to do with me! That's the "Jürgen dirt." (Jürgen is a colleague from the client's sports association.)
Therapist: I see, this mucus actually belongs to Jürgen. Maybe you can imagine a huge sieve or filter which, when you are ready, you can pass through and, with that, everything you no longer want. Everything that doesn't belong to you, including the Jürgen dirt, gets stuck. Take your time, only you know what this sieve, filter, or whatever else fits right now, must look like.
Client: Yes, it is a huge curtain.
Therapist: Let me know when you're ready to go through that curtain to get rid of all that mucus and everything that doesn't belong to you.
Client: I'm ready.

> *Therapist:*   Now take a deep breath. Yes, exactly, and while exhaling –
> shshshsh – you move through the curtain!
>
> The client exhales and adopts the "shshsh" noise of the therapist.
>
> *Client:*   It's better now, lighter.
> *Therapist:*   Where do you feel it?
> *Client:*   Mainly in my belly, it feels normal now.

This section of the therapy shows how the healthy self-assertive power of anger can be extracted and separated from the real and unchangeable stresses from the outer world. The suggestion with the sieve, along the lines of Emmerson's *Separation Sieve* (2014), facilitates liberating oneself from imposed burdens, thus promoting a liberating active boundary experience. Of course, in real life, the hostility of the grousers will not stop due to this intervention, yet the client experiences correction on the inner stage, not only lightening up his "gut feeling" but also improving his ability to cope with the challenges of the next session in the sports association. Since this did not solve the problem, we completed the therapy session with *sentences of self-acceptance* and an exercise of self-regulation to empower him for the meeting at the sports association. Later, the client reported that though the meeting at the association had been very strenuous, it had gone off without a hitch.

In the past, clients were often not allowed to get angry, or it was not possible or too dangerous for them to do so. The dialogue with introjects on the inner stage not only offers a corrective experience, but also the possibility, along the lines of Emmerson's "Introject Speak" (2014), to disengage from interdictions of the past and, if desired, to reconcile with prohibiting authorities.

> A female client suffers from a bad conscience when she gets angry in everyday life situations and therefore, she finds it difficult to allow for her anger, though she wishes she were allowed to be angry. When the therapist asks her to immerse herself in a typical situation, the client feels a wave of anger, at the same time sensing fear, warm and cold, running through her entire body from the bottom up and paralyzing her.
>
> *Therapist:*   How old do you feel?
> *Client:*   12 or 13 years old.
>
> Therapist May I speak to the 12/13-year-old? Yes? What may I call her?

Client as Sandra:	I actually want to be angry but can't move. The fear stops me from expressing my anger.
Therapist:	Where are you, Sandra?
Client:	At home.
Therapist:	Is somebody with you?
Client:	I'm alone.
Therapist:	Why can't you be angry?
Client:	Because they won't love me anymore. Then I'll be even more alone.

The therapist explains to the client that this is not happening now, that it is over and that she now has the power and possibility to change the situation so she can be angry and still part of the community, something she would have been entitled to be already back then. Thereupon, Sandra assembles her whole family outside on the lawn, shouting and stamping her feet with anger in the midst of them, like Rumpelstiltskin, the other children joining her. However, Sandra is still afraid when she sees the critical looks from the adults, especially her mother.

Subsequently Sandra speaks to her mother on her inner stage. Through this intervention the anger is uncoupled from the fear of being expelled from the community. Thanks to the dialogue with her inner mother, "Sandra" gets permission to be angry, so that from now on the grownup client can be angry without the fear of the young ego state "Sandra" being triggered by the implicit interdiction of the mother introject. Such inner dialogues with important attachment figures from childhood can resolve and readjust many issues even if in reality a settlement is not possible because the attachment figure is dead, or the relationship is not safe enough, or the necessary preconditions are missing. The more stressed or difficult the relationship to the person is, the more carefully this dialogue needs to be prepared and accompanied. The therapist can then check with the client whether they are ready for this step. In case of *rejection*, as above (it does not matter whether the rejection was real, what matters is only the experience, the reaction of the client), Emmerson (2014) recommends the "Introject Speak," that is, a dialogue with the introject takes place, where you work with chairs, inviting the client to alternate between sitting on one chair and then the other. The purpose of putting oneself in the position of the parent figures is to develop understanding and empathy for them. Clients begin to understand that they were rejected because the mother or father could not act otherwise, they were in distress, or not able to accept their child the way they were, the problem being with the attachment figure and not with *them*. As soon as the clients have returned to their own chair again, the therapist can ask the child part: Do you understand now that you are absolutely lovable the way you are and that the rejection does not have to do with you but with X (the parent)?

A 24-year-old client wants to overcome his fear of migraine, which is associated with many compulsive acts. He would like to "accept" the migraine and uncouple it from the compulsion. The fear of migraine is most threatening during exams or when having to write a term paper.

The therapist asks him to remember a specific situation in which this fear surfaced. When he has found a situation, she asks him to close his eyes and "enter" the situation.

Client:	We examinees are waiting in front of the hall, and now we go inside and I take my seat.
Therapist:	What do you feel?
Client:	There is a feeling of constriction and fear in the lower chest area. I keep having to look around, controlling my sight (*beginning of an aura constricting sight, a prodrome of the migraine*), by looking around. I'm afraid of losing control.
Therapist:	What else do you notice?
Client:	Irritation. It's so unfair!
Therapist:	Where in your body do you feel this irritation?
Client:	In the elbows. There is also the fear of not being taken seriously.
Therapist:	Stay with these feelings and sensations for a moment.
Client:	I'm feeling dizzy.

The therapist asks the client to stand up and gives him a set of batakas (swords made of foam rubber with solid hilts), asking:

Therapist:	What's that like?
Client:	My arms and upper body are covered with anger.

The therapist invites him to project his anger into the batakas and to lightly swing his arms. The client starts swinging the batakas tentatively. The therapist supports him

Therapist:	Yes, exactly!

The therapist also swings her arms back and forth vigorously, exhaling with a noisy "ha" when lowering her arms.

After a few swinging movements, she invites the client to rest and to sense what it is like now.

Client:	I feel relaxed and not so much filled with anger anymore.

After five or six vigorous swinging movements, the therapist asks the client to pause again.

Client:	Now I feel even more relaxation.
Therapist:	Where do you feel that?
Client:	In my fingers. The elbows are also more relaxed.

After the third round, the Client now swinging his arms with ever more power and at the same time with more ease in his shoulders, accompanied by a strong exhale, reports: The anger has now dropped and is more neutral. My arms feel light. I'm not so much at the mercy of the anger anymore.

Therapist:	So now . . .?
Client:	I can decide what to do with my anger. . . .
Therapist:	What's that like?
Client:	It gives me a sense of control, of being more on top of it.
Therapist:	Where do you feel that?
Client:	In my lower legs and shoulders. There is solidity there.
Therapist:	Have you had enough of the swinging?

The client says yes and sits back down on his chair.

Therapist:	What's it like now?
Client:	There's still a small fear I might get attacked by a migraine, like in a house that isn't locked. It's a feeling of being at its mercy.
Therapist:	How old do you feel?
Client:	Sixteen years old.
Therapist:	What may I call you? Who are you, feeling at the mercy?
Client:	I'm the part who had to go to hospital with a sudden hemiplegia (*which was later diagnosed as his first migraine attack*).
Therapist:	What may I call you?
Client:	Powerless.
Therapist:	Powerless, where are you? Are you in a building or outside?
Client:	I'm in a changing room after PE. My mates and myself notice that something is wrong. (The client turns pale.)
Therapist:	Powerless, this is not happening to you now. It is over. It is a memory, a memory you can change now. You now have the power to change everything in a way that is good for you. And you know that in your imagination everything is possible. What is important now so you do not need to feel so powerless anymore?
Client:	I'd like to get out of the building. I need somebody to carry me.
Therapist:	Who could do that?
Client:	My grandmother!
Therapist:	Where does she take you?
Client:	To a magician who can heal me, no, he can make it undone!

Therapist:	How does he do that?
Client:	With a spell.
Therapist:	What's it like now, Powerless?
Client:	I can observe my body. I can fully stand now. The paresthesia in the hand is disappearing, the left half of my face is no longer hanging down, I can speak again!
Therapist:	What's that like?
Client:	I feel strong again!
Therapist:	Where do you feel this strength?
Client:	In my upper arms.
Therapist:	Wonderful! Keep your attention on your upper arms for a moment! (She gives him time.) What's it like now?
Client:	I feel bigger.
Therapist:	Does the name Powerless still fit?
Client:	No.
Therapist:	What may I call you now?
Client:	Healed.
Therapist:	Healed, I'm so happy. Do you understand that it is over and that you are healed? Do you still need anything now?
Client:	Yes, the magician could also give me a protection spell.
Therapist:	Very good. Let it happen and give me a sign when the protection spell's effect is strong enough. (He gives a sign.) Thank you for talking to me, Healed. I am now talking to you again, what's it like for you now?
Client:	I'm relieved that I do not have to worry anymore!

When confronted with his fear of losing control, the client experiences anger and powerlessness at the same time, as well as dizziness. However, the anger seems to be stuck and can only be felt in the elbows. To bring the client out of the freeze into movement, the therapist asks him to stand up. Because she does not have Smovie rings, she gives him batakas with solid hilts that he can grasp, so he can channel his anger. With the therapist's guidance he can start moving. It is important for the client to keep pausing, to feel what is happening, noticing his sensations and naming them. The client starts moving, supported by a strong exhale. His feelings change pretty quickly from powerlessness to control and self-determination. If the therapist is not sure whether or not more is needed, they can ask the client whether it feels like enough. By sensing into it the client knows exactly what is needed and when the physical corrective experience is complete.

Conflicted Ego States – The Inner Dilemma

Sometimes clients feel immense anger on one hand, but at the same time another ego state can emerge putting on the brake and not allowing the anger to be expressed. In this case it can be helpful to let the client choose a chair for each of these parts, allowing the client to sit on each chair respectively and express what is being felt there, so both can have their say and are respected and considered. It is not necessary to find a solution or for both parts to agree immediately. The fact that both can express themselves is, in and of itself, a relief, and is relaxing for the client. The therapist acts as a presenter who supports the conflicting ego states to listen and respect each other and express themselves, by appreciating both of them so they can start negotiating.

Exploring the Root of Violence

With violent clients or those directing their anger in real life at the outer world, the approach is different. Here, clients are asked to pause just before striking and to sense what it feels like. That is, they are invited to show how they would execute the aggressive act, how they would strike, but before actually doing the aggressive movement, they are stopped by the therapist and urged to remain in the body posture just before striking, to notice their sensations and to name them. Should this posture be too frightening or overwhelming (for client or therapist), it may also be imagined with similar results. By freezing the act, the client can perceive the feelings that were fended off behind this violent action, i.e., covered up by the aggressive act because they are too painful. If these feelings are given space and attention respectfully, be it only for a short moment – that is, if the violent anger is uncoupled from the painful underlying emotions – this often results in tears releasing what was held back for a long time (Levine, 2017). Anger and disgust often serve as a defense against shame. More about this later.

   As another option, the client may be invited to clench his fist tightly and to wait and see what happens. Eventually his hand will start to release and open and the client is encouraged to just observe what happens.

Refernces

Emmerson, G. (2014): *Resource Therapy. The Complete Guide with Case Examples & Transcripts.* Victoria: Old Golden Point.

Levine, P. (2017): Shame and Pride, Seminar in Weggis, Switzerland (12–15 August 2017).

Paulsen, S. (2009): *Looking through the Eyes of Trauma and Dissociation. An Illustrated Guide for EMDR Therapists and Clients.* BookSurge Publishing.

Watkins, H. H. (1980): The Silent Abreaction. *The International Journal of Clinical and Experimental Hypnosis, 28*: 101–113.

Chapter **6**

Shame and Guilt

Shame, the Hidden Emotion

Shame is an extremely painful and powerful human emotion, present in all humans and mammals, across all cultures. It has a central influence on life. Shame determines the emotional mood of a person more than sexuality or aggression. Although shame is so vital, people are either not aware of it or they keep it concealed or secret. Shame is everywhere and yet it is only marginally considered when dealing with feelings (Marks, 2016). On the one hand, there is little research on shame; on the other, shame is often mistaken for fear, anger, or disgust. All pathologies associated with self-condemnation or self-devaluation have to do with shame.

Shame is closely related to trauma. The particular body posture and autonomic pattern of shame are similar to those of trauma (Levine, 2017). When treating trauma, shame should also be considered, disentangled, and resolved. Therapists should respect vulnerable people with shame and realize how easily they can be shamed (again) und how carefully this issue should be approached. In fact, shame is often ignored although it is sitting in the therapy room like a gorilla weighing 300 kilos. If shame is not treated, it spreads like cancer and is passed on to later generations (Levine, 2017). Yet – whoever is without shame also lacks empathy and does not care for other people, and that is dangerous.

Cultural factors, such as social norms, religion, the legacy of ancestors, passed on over many generations – on multiple levels, including epigenetically – play a fundamental role in the way shame is formed. In societies with many moral rules, there is a high level of shame. Shame is all about dominance and submission. Shame is used to powerfully establish and implement rigid social structures. Levine (2017) describes shame as a "glue of loyalty." Everything is done in order not to be expelled from the community. It is exactly the same with primates (Levine, 2017).

Polyvagal theory (Levine, 2017) furnishes the following explanation: In so-called shame cultures there is little "ventral" contact, the type of contact from which the social engagement system develops, meaning, holding and cradling the infant is not supported. Even in the last century, the Swiss pediatrician and pioneer of pediatrics, Marie Meierhofer, was treated with hostility, because she postulated

DOI: 10.4324/9781003460602-7

that crying babies should be picked up and held. Parents who were not picked up and held as babies pass on this *neglect* to the next generation. As a result of missing physical contact or suffering a total rupture in contact, they have internalized deep feelings of shame associated with being "unworthy" or "insignificant."

Holding and cradling a baby leads to safety, tickling to pleasant excitement whilst at the same time *remaining in contact*, and can be found in all cultures. It promotes *shared joy and warmth*. Children experiencing a lot of joy and having many pleasant experiences are more resilient and less prone to pathological or toxic shame (Levine, 2017).

Feelings of shame can range from feeling embarrassed, inhibited, or shy to overall agonizing self-doubt, where the individual feels exposed and vulnerable. Shame is disabling, cutting back people's vitality and making them feel stuck. You can feel ashamed of yourself, of others or of the community, such as the family or nation. Shame can be healthy and natural or take over the whole personality in a toxic way and become chronic.

Marks (2016) proposes different forms of shame: The *shame of adaptation* relates to oneself and gets triggered by the presumption that one is not conforming to the prevailing expectations or standards of the collective. It provides conformity with the expectations of the group. Every family or society depends on their members sticking to the norms. Learning these norms is associated with natural feelings of adaptation shame. A two-year-old boy sticking his finger in his brother's eye and then being reprimanded by his parents will react with shamefaced frustration, avert his eyes, and start weeping bitterly. For the rule, "Don't stick your finger in somebody's eyes, to be internalized, a strong stimulus is needed. An overwhelming feeling of shame does the trick. If the parents intimate to the infant that its *behavior* and not the child as a *person* is unacceptable, then shame has fulfilled its function of adaptation and remains healthy. However, if the child is rejected as a person or punished with breaking off contact, the shame becomes pathological. For parents, there is a fine line between setting clear boundaries and instilling shame. In mammals, shame plays the same important role. It stops behavior that is threatening for the tribe. A defiant young elephant is immediately reprimanded loudly and encircled by its aunts, whereupon it responds with a submissive demeanor. In Porges' terminology, shame is a parasympathetic brake.

Another form of shame is *group shame* (*vicarious embarrassment*), which relates to other people. You can be ashamed of a mentally ill family member, for example. With group shame, you take distance from a member of your own community who is doing wrong, or are perceived in this way, no longer feeling solidarity with the individual threatening the group. Adaptation shame and group shame are mechanisms of social control.

Empathic shame, yet another form, is also directed at other people. We sympathize when we witness how another human is being shamed. It enables us to sense the feelings of shame others have, allowing us to feel connection and solidarity with the other.

Intimacy shame protects our privacy towards others, thus enabling us to keep our own boundaries. We do not tell everybody our most secret affairs. Obviously, these boundaries have shifted with the use of social media.

When an individual's privacy or boundaries have been grossly violated by others, such as with sexual abuse or violence, *traumatic shame* occurs. The ability to protect oneself in a healthy manner is lost or impaired. This results in excessive protective behavior or the inability to protect oneself.

With *conscience shame* a person feels ashamed of their behavior not conforming with their own conscience or the necessary respect for another person. As a result of their conscience shame, the person realizes their fault and that they have to apologize. Thus, this form of shame protects the person's integrity regarding their own moral values. As with adaptation shame, the ethical principles of the group, the collective conscience, are thus internalized. From an ego state perspective, one or more "inner critic" states are generated when shame is internalized. With a healthy adaptation shame, these remain valuable and necessary self-critical parts of the personality, whereas with a pathological traumatic shame, these inner critics keep devaluing the person. But not only that, young injured states still believe the messages of the critics in the present and are convinced of their own worthlessness.

Often there are other parts trying to avoid shame. These turn to problematic behavior such as addiction, self-harming, or aggression, triggering even more embarrassment and shame. Especially when it comes to sexual abuse in childhood, clients and their young ego states are convinced that they are responsible and could have prevented it from happening, feeling deeply ashamed about it. In therapy, *differentiating* between ones' own shame and being put to shame by others is important, as can be seen in the case study of the 64-year-old female client described next. However, it is usually not enough to talk about it, the person must also experience it. A good way to access this is to work with the opposite poles of shame and dignity in the way described.

How do we experience shame? We feel assaulted, surprised, and the experienced loss of self-control makes us feel powerless, worthless – and actually devastated. There is a sense of helplessness, of annihilation, non-existence, of being gutted. Levine emphasizes that the organism reacts to a large extent autonomously and he speaks of a typical shame posture. As with trauma, there is a collapse. People who are feeling ashamed will lower and turn their head, interrupting eye contact, or not focusing their gaze, their eyes darting in all directions, their shoulders dropping forward, as they blush and sweat. Sometimes you can see the person's facial muscles drooping, as the person turns pale, their pupils contracting.

People sometimes report nausea, dizziness, or buzzing in their ears. The subjective experience of shame is always very strong. Reactions are similar to those seen in trauma. Levine (2017) refers to an MRI study: When showing a test subject an image of a friendly face, their prefrontal cortex is activated. The person is interpreted as benevolent and safe. Yet if the same face is shown to a traumatized person in the same collapsed state as with an experience of shame, the frontal lobe becomes inactive and the periaqueductal gray in the brainstem lights up. This is the part of the brainstem associated with fight/flight or freeze/immobility responses (Lanius et al., 2002). In dealing with trauma and shame, therapists tend to fall into a trap. They see that the client is ashamed and try to be friendly and supportive to make the person feel better. However, if you bear in mind this study, it becomes apparent that these efforts are of no avail. Quite the contrary, the client is put to shame all the more, feeling even more helpless and worthless, because they can hardly tolerate eye contact. van der Kolk (2017) also emphasizes how omnipresent shame is in chronic traumatization.

In posttraumatic disorders, not the actual event, but self-reproaches and shame are the main problem — the relationship of the individual to his or her inner self.
(van der Kolk, Video 7, Part 1)

van der Kolk suggests differentiating clearly between the client of today and the child back then, thus enabling corrective experiences on the inner stage, as is common practice in Ego State therapy. But not only that, van der Kolk (2017) recommends working in three-dimensional space because then you can switch from linear, left hemisphere thinking to the spatial, non-verbal emotionality of the right hemisphere where shame resides.

In deep shame, the right hemisphere is activated to the point of feeling existential fear or fear of death. The organism tries to get away from the fear and has three possibilities of shame control: *Freeze, flight, or fight.* Freezing manifests through hiding and withdrawal; you just want the ground to open up and swallow you, you stay stuck in the pain, tense, unable to act, often followed by a deep sadness. Porges (in Buczynski, 2017) suggests asking clients where they feel the shame in their body. When there is freezing, the reaction always occurs below the diaphragm, similar to when there is a life-threatening situation. The person wants to disappear, not wanting to be present, and that leads to dissociation and collapse. The autonomous functions of the organism take over and deliberate control is no longer possible, leading to immobility. When clients feel shame, they freeze, turn away, and are no longer in contact with the therapist.

What can therapists do? If the therapist can move the client to act deliberately, asking the person to stand up, to breathe in a certain way, to make a gesture, the sympathetic nervous system is activated through this deliberate movement, inhibiting the dorsal-vagal immobility reaction (Porges in Buczynski, 2017). In order to come out of a state of shame, movement or at least a change of body posture is necessary, something Levine also emphasizes.

Flight impulses cause breaking away from the shame-related situation, like taking refuge in delusions of grandeur, idealization, perfectionism, or addiction. With the *fight reaction* you switch to counter attacking: You become angry, aggressive, or arrogant towards other people or fend off shame through contempt, cynicism, negativity, shamelessness, arrogance, defiance, rage, or anger to the point of violence. In certain cultures, this is reflected by restoring one's honor. However, the impulse to punish the person who has put us to shame and shame them for their part, so as to take revenge, exists in all societies.

Shame happens in relationships to others, involving the ventral vagal system of social engagement: You feel ashamed in front of somebody. You withhold your aggression towards the other person as well as your fear of not being able to regulate it. Usually, you try to hide your shame, which makes you feel even worse, but if the shame can be repaired and corrected, this leads to strengthening and triumph.

Healthy Shame – Toxic Shame

Chronic shame is the root of all evil in the world.

(Levine, 2017)

The precursors of shame already develop in the first few months of our lives: Child and mother or the caretaker communicate through eye and body contact. The baby has open eyes, searching, as Kohut says, for a shine in the eye of its parents reflecting love (Marks, 2016). According to Erik Erikson's (1950) psychosocial developmental phases of the personality, either a basic trust or mistrust in life develops through this interaction in the first 18 months. In Levine's view (2017), early shame emotions begin at the age of about 15 months when a new neurotransmitter system starts developing, the dopamine system. It is related to gratification and high levels of activation. At that age, babies explore everything in their environment. Therefore, they must be stopped and prevented, as effectively as possible, from behavior that is dangerous for them. At the same time, the baby should be able to internalize this "no" as a rule, also for the future, so it must be connected to a strong emotion inhibiting the whole organism, which, for Levine, is the explanation and reason for the intensity of the shame reaction. Erik Erikson called this developmental phase between the first and the third year "autonomy versus shame."

However, if the infant is stopped without its needs being met, self-doubts develop, and shame becomes toxic. With agitated shame, the baby tries to defend against it and the sympathetic nervous system and the dorsal vagus are activated, whereas with collapsed shame, there is a dorsal vagal collapse. The "real" emotion of shame only develops at the age of about three-and-a-half years, feelings of guilt even later (see Table 6.1). Though shame is one root of guilt, its origin is much more primitive, because in shame, the reptilian brain and the limbic system are involved, in guilt also the frontal cortex.

How can shame stay healthy and functional? For parents, there is a fine line between setting boundaries and suffocating the child's curiosity. Boundaries, containment, and restraint are necessary, and therefore the parent's reactions are so important. The rule or boundary must be internalized, but not in a way that is overwhelming and leading to collapse. If parents break off their contact to the infant, there is a "vacuum" that is filled with shame (Levine, 2017), so it is vital to keep the *connection* when setting boundaries. If, on the other hand, parents do not set boundaries, the child reacts with anger, because their needs are not respected, amounting to neglect. Hidden behind the anger are also shame and sadness. On the one hand, *anger* is a way of defending against shame, but on the other hand it activates the *courage* badly needed to confront the feelings of shame. So, anger can cover up the shame but also lead to liberation and victory.

For Levine (2017), anger and also disgust are "door openers" for shame in therapy. In its original function, *disgust* prevents us from eating poisonous food, making us spit it out. So, seen from this angle, disgust is a self-protection and defense reaction of the organism. When differentiated and uncoupled from other emotions, such as fear, disgust usually disappears completely.

People with cynophobia are often disgusted by the animals' saliva. When these people are exposed to real dogs, in order to learn to handle their anxiety, and are invited to feed them, they feel fear and disgust. These two emotions can easily be uncoupled by first noticing the disgust without trying to change it: It is okay to feel disgusted by the dog's saliva and that doesn't have to change. You only want to reduce the fear to a normal degree of respect. Then the therapist invites the client to put on a rubber glove, thus eliminating the disgust, and focusing on overcoming the fear. Interestingly enough, the disgust disappears in most cases as soon as the fear has been overcome. The clients then feed the dogs without gloves (Zanotta, 2013).

With shame, the child has also been forced to swallow something that does not agree with them. *Anger* as well as *disgust* help to *spit out shame again*. Disgust may also help to get rid of the internalized abashing voices. In working with disgust, it is therefore necessary to stay with this unpleasant emotion until it can fulfill its natural function.

In the therapy section with Ms. Y in Chapter 1, the client accepts the disgust, allowing it to exist without wanting to change it or get rid of it. She recognizes that, in its original function, the disgust is a defense reaction and protection, and uncouples it from the fear behind it, that is, the state overwhelmed with fear that developed in the preverbal phase.

On closer inspection, violence also often stems from shame and abashment. Furthermore, Levine speaks about narcissism and borderline symptoms being "driven by shame." Narcissists react to abashment with indignation and protest, defending themselves vehemently. They will not allow anyone to pass criticism on their person, so are obviously caught in an aroused or even angry mode of shame, whereas a person with borderline symptoms remains in a collapsed shame, in destructive feelings of powerlessness and the existential fear of being abandoned. These people oscillate between auto-aggressive self-hatred on the one hand, and the projection of shame onto others by means of aggression and degradation on the other, so they do not have to feel this awful state.

To support corrective experiences in therapy, the therapist must realize what an infant in these sensitive phases of development needs. The parents need to be **reliable**, **loving** and respectful of the **child's boundaries**, so a healthy sense of self-worth, as well as healthy intimacy, shame, and dignity may develop. Dignity means: *I am lovable and I can protect my boundaries.*

If, however, this early communication is defective, the sense of self-worth is compromised and results in traumatic shame. This is the most painful, destructive, and debilitating of all feelings: *I am unworthy of being, I am an object, nothing, worthless and I am* **existentially threatened**. This activates the primal fear of being expelled from the collective, which would entail death without fail. The experience of being shamed is absorbed and turns into self-shaming, leading to the primal shame of being unloved (Marks, 2016).

With sexual abuse, the child experiences itself as an object of satisfaction for the needs of others. To resolve this terrible situation, the dilemma between being dependent on attachment and needing autonomy, in other words, realizing its own needs, the child internalizes a primal shame: I am not worth it, I do not deserve it. The child is ashamed of its existence. In addition, the child begins to feel guilty . . . If I had acted in such a way, this would not have happened. I provoked it. Maybe even wanted it?

When the parents suffer from depression or addiction, the child's needs are also not met and the child feels worthless and ashamed. Under these circumstances, the roles are switched with parentification being the manifestation. The children try to take care of the parents by being as adaptable, reasonable, or caring as possible – at a high cost. They are unable to cope, which in turn amplifies the shame and the feeling of being ashamed: *I am incapable.*

Shame versus Guilt

Table 6.1 shows that shame is a feeling that usually occurs with socially undesirable characteristics or modes of behavior, especially when these are unmasked or discovered. Shame is an alarm signal indicating that an individual's affiliation to a group is endangered when the behavior or character deviates too much from the prevailing norms. When implicit social rules are violated and witnessed by other members of the group, the individual is in danger of being excluded from the group. The control rests with an external authority. However, feelings of guilt require higher cognitive functions because they relate to internalized ideals. They arise when a person becomes aware of having made a mistake. This mistake does not concern the person as a whole and can be admitted and repaired. Here, the controlling authority has been internalized, residing within the person (Marks, 2016).

Shame and guilt are biologically useful feelings, protecting peaceful cooperation in a group. Yet both feelings can become dysfunctional when they meet unrealistically high expectations or standards that cannot be met. This results in chronic guilt or shame, which only disappear when the self-concepts that are unrealistic or the introjects of the perpetrator are corrected. A deeply felt "basic shame" is devastating: One feels "wrong" and worthless as a whole person.

Table. 6.1 Differentiating among shame, healthy and unhealthy guilt, based on Buczynski, R. (2017) and Marks (2016)

Shame	Helpful, "healthy" guilt	Not helpful, "unhealthy" guilt
Feeling: I am worthless, wrong, I am a mistake.	Fact: I have done something wrong.	Feeling of having done something wrong due to unrealistic expectations.
Controlling external authority. Feelings of shame due to abashment.	Controlling internal authority. Twinges of remorse due to punishment.	Controlling internal authority. Twinges of remorse due to unrealistic expectations.
Thomas has the feeling of being absolutely worthless, nothing but a burden and a waste of time.	Leo was drunk and hit somebody with the car and feels guilty.	Patricia has forgotten the name of one of her colleagues at work and feels guilty because of that.
In a monologue: Withdrawal into oneself.	In a dialogue: Relating to the person injured.	In a dialogue: Twinges of remorse related to the supposedly injured person.
Developmentally early, starting at 15 months. Therefore, the shame is more deeply rooted and more resistant to therapy.	Developmentally late, starting at age three to six years. Requires a more mature development of the brain.	Developmentally late, starting at age three to six years.
Effect: Negative	Effect: Positive	Effect: Negative
"Unshaming" not possible	Development of conscience.	Leads to self-punishment and being caught in guilt instead of change of behavior.
Exception: Healthy conscience shame leading to remorse: "In the future, I will act differently."	Exculpation possible: Realizing fault, pleading guilty and/or reparation is healing.	
Treatment:	Treatment:	Treatment:
Focus on dignity and pride, self-acceptance. Building and facilitating human relationships in order to experience belonging.	Acknowledging fault, taking charge, offering an excuse, changing destructive behavior, reparation.	Differentiating between healthy and unhealthy guilt, resolving unhealthy guilt.
On the inner stage: Ego State therapy, self-acceptance, tapping.	On the inner stage: Ego State therapy.	Self-acceptance: I accept my strengths and weaknesses.
		Supporting connection with others.
		On the inner stage: Ego State therapy, self-acceptance, tapping.

Thus, shame and guilt are not the same. If we understand the difference between the two, they can more easily be uncoupled, and the self-degradation and negative self-concepts associated with them can more easily be changed. Guilt can be healthy or unhealthy. Unhealthy guilt may be implanted by others, by destructive introjects, and is therefore toxic.

Dealing Constructively with Shame, Repairing Shame

"Do not despise those who helped you when you were in trouble," said the king to the princess, when she refused to go to bed with the Frog King (Grimm, 2012). Out of rage, she threw him against the wall, whereupon he turned into a prince.

The issue of shame can be found in many fairytales, such as Cinderella, the Frog King, and Iron Henry, occurring in combination with all the emotions that can cover up shame, including anger, fear, and disgust. What actually *happens* with the shame in those fairy tales? How do the protagonists find their way out of it? Let's take the Frog King as an example. The princess does not want the frog, she avoids it anxiously, feeling disgusted and shamed by it. It is only when she allows herself to disobey her father and casts the frog against the wall in anger, thus switching from passive avoidance to active coping and defense, that the true nature of the ugly frog shows itself in the shape of a handsome prince. The shaming situation is only resolved once she actually confronts it.

Levine (2017) advises us to recognize shame, presenting as vulnerability in the physiology of the clients, as a reflection of their family history, against the background of the culture in which their ancestors lived. Like the princess with the frog,

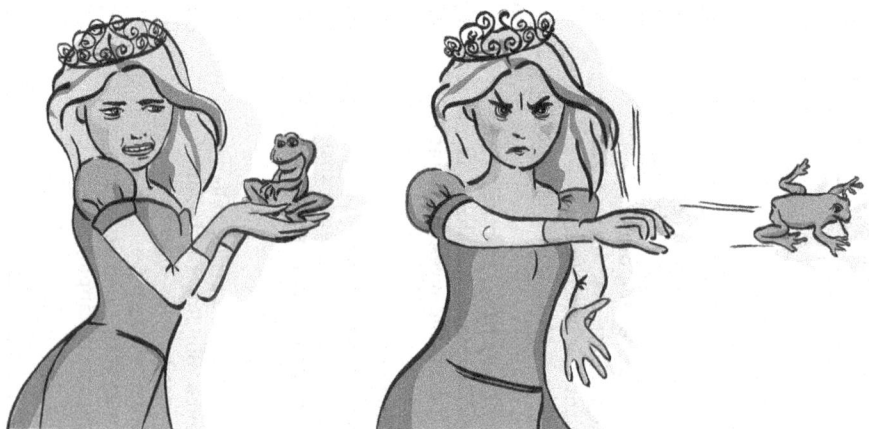

Figure 6.1 The Princess and the Frog – Disgust and anger

the client is afraid of the devastating feelings of shame, trying by all means to avoid and ignore them. Thus, the shame remains hidden.

The first step is to recognize shame as such and to face it. How can I discern shame from other feelings and perceive it accurately? How and what can I utilize it for? What kind of shame is it? What kind of behavior does this feeling want to induce?

To support clients in facing shame, therapists can help them recognize and appreciate their particular defense against shame as a useful defense strategy of the past, and then to transform it into an adequate protection, not separating them from others but rather allowing for connection. Rather than excluding the "problem" part, the defense against shame can be appreciated and seen as protector of a vulnerable and precious side of the individual. Clients can be helped to discover the hidden treasure behind the defense, or the prince in the character of the frog.

Connection not Destruction

Experts such as Porges, Siegel, and van der Kolk, all agree that in dealing with shame we need to focus on a healthy authentic therapeutic relationship (Buczynski, 2017). Only when feeling safely accompanied and supported by the connection to the therapist can the client approach difficult and dangerous feelings such as shame, cautiously and in small steps. In addition to safety and acceptance, people dealing with shame need the connection to another human being. For this, touch can be essential so the client can actually experience the connection. The couple therapist Bill O'Hanlon invites couples to support each other with touch in situations involving shame (Buczynski, 2017). Levine, positioned next to his clients, touches the upper arm or shoulder of his clients very softly and lightly to help them tolerate difficult feelings when they show up, suggesting and letting them feel: "I am here, and I will stay here, even in these difficult moments."

As described, loyalty plays an important role when handling shame, which is why it is important to build a connection and loyalty to oneself: I remain true to myself and yet functional within society.

Levine also emphasizes working with the *attitude* of shame. As shown by Nina Bull in her classic work (Bull, 1962), the feelings of the people tested did not change unless they also changed their attitude. Again, the exact knowledge of the actual content of the experience is not so relevant, because self-condemnation, involving shame dissolves when the attitude, including the physiological pattern, is shifted. The submissive physiognomy of shame must gradually be transformed into a dominant alpha physiognomy of *healthy self-assertion*. Deep shame equals collapse and total loss of energy, and is accompanied by feelings of helplessness and hopelessness, powerlessness and immobility. As soon as clients move out of this position they begin to feel more alive, lighter and better, allowing for the opposite pole of shame to surface: Dignity, joy, and triumph. Dignity signifies: *I am lovable and I can respect my boundaries*. It is best to first explore this opposite pole with the client in a standing position, carefully inquiring into body sensations, feelings, and thoughts it involves, and then to reinforce it:

> "What do you enjoy? . . . What makes you enthusiastic? . . . What do you feel when you talk about that? . . . How does that feel in your body? . . . Take your time to know more about this joy, enjoy it for as long as you like . . . !"
>
> "How do you experience dignity? What happens when you imagine dignity? What is dignity for you?"
>
> "With severely depressive clients: What change would you most wish for? What makes you go on, what enables you to continue living? Is there something bigger than you? What do you feel when you think of this presence? Where in your body do you feel this power?"

After having explored this carefully, Levine (2017) suggests inviting the client to move in one way or another, using questions such as:

> "Can you express this joy with your body, with a movement? What would be an appropriate posture?"
>
> Then, therapist and client perform this movement together several times or adopt the body posture mentioned, the therapist then asking the client to pause:
>
> "Very good! And now, rest for a moment and notice how your body reacts to these movements, to this posture!"

For people who have experienced a lot of repression, joy is a banned emotion, covered up by shame which acts as a lid, making sure it remains suppressed: You should not exist!

It is not necessary to bring movement into play, yet devices such as rings (Smovie Rings), batakas (swords made of foam), the Bellicon (trampoline), or tuning boards[1], used in the treatment of trauma with Somatic Experiencing®, can serve as catalysts. Only after having carefully explored and established the body sensations, postures, movements, and thoughts associated with joy, does the therapist invite the client to make two steps to the side to switch to the bad feeling of shame.

> "What happens when you think of the word shame? . . . Are you ready to find out a bit more about your shame? . . . How do you feel doing so? . . . Where do you feel it?"

The therapist must pay attention that the client does not remain in a position of shame for too long and is not overwhelmed by these destructive feelings. Often clients have blockages in the shoulder area. You can invite them to join you in an experiment, softly swinging your arms and just trying out what that movement feels like, leading them from freeze into movement. If the area of the jaw and mouth are tense you can ask them to imagine biting into an apple:

> "Here is a delicious apple. Slowly take a bite and taste the apple in your mouth, chewing it slowly. Is it sweet? . . . When you swallow it, really absorb it into your body."

For the experience to be truly corrective, it is vital not only to bring in movement but also to establish a connection.

> "Look around! Take in this feeling of connection with your environment through your eyes!"

Then you can ask your client to stand in the place of joy.

The client willingly enters the shame-posture and moves out again. The key to liberation from shame is this self-directed back and forth.

With shame, the trick is to move in and out, then the underlying emotions and body reactions become evident. The longer this in and out is possible, the more likely you will reach the root of the shame (Levine, 2017).

You pendulate between shame and dignity, always remaining at the periphery of the trauma and the counter vortex. The state of dignity can also be called joy, triumph, or pride, whatever fits (Levine, 2017). It is best to work standing – therapist and client – and to place yourself next to them, accompanying them by matching their pace and co-regulating. The advantage of standing is that it is easier for clients to initiate movement, it helps them come out of freezing, making it easier to clearly take the positions of both poles and feeling them. You can ask them to take a step to the side when they switch from one state to another, so they are standing in different places for the different states, then have them switch back and forth between the two places. After having pendulated between the two positions for a while, the therapist can ask the client in their position of dignity what they would like to say to the shame-part, and the dignity part can explain to the part that was ashamed back then: "This experience does not last, others shamed you and that shame does not belong to you." Or the dignity part can even express that it is proud of the shamed part and its stamina.

Many clients express sentences like these spontaneously, others need support from the therapist. Then, clients can be invited to go back to the same position again and to notice what they feel now. Often, the younger parts that used to be ashamed feel touched once they realize that the shame has fallen off them in favor of more strength, expansion, and growth. Again, it is important to give these states plenty of acknowledgment and compassion. However, compassion should not be overemphasized as they may begin to feel they are receiving too much, becoming overwhelmed and therefore ashamed again.

A 64-year-old woman, now radiating with a beautiful smile, was bullied as a child because of her braces, which she had to wear for over seven years. At the time, the protocol was excruciating, and she had to see the dentist weekly, suffering from toothache and not being able to eat for days. She was harassed, insulted, and called "horse-toothed" by the other children for many years. Feeling deeply abashed, she tried not to show the braces, and even when smiling, took care not to uncover her upper incisors.

The therapist invites her to stand up and pick two spots, one suitable for the state of dignity and one for the state of shame. First, she is asked to enter the spot of dignity, and to take the time to feel it in her body. Outside the window, she sees a swan on a lake. This swan has dignity, she says, thus spontaneously contacting her own dignity: She describes a state of growth, feeling upright and dignified, "like a swan." The therapist explores with her all the body sensations, thoughts, images, and the body posture involved. The therapist listens in an understanding way and encourages the client over and over to observe what is happening in her body, thus establishing with her this state of dignity to the point where the client clearly notices her body sensations and can describe them (integration and stabilization). The client spreads out her arms, feeling more and more expansion. Her left arm is quite relaxed, the right one seems rather tense, as if locked. She describes: It doesn't quite come along with the left one and doesn't know where to go. The client reports that she had broken her right wrist six months earlier.

Therapist: Could the left arm somehow help the right one?
Client: Yes, the two just have to come together, the right lower arm wants to be held. She brings her hands together in front of her chest and starts stroking her right wrist and hand, as if putting on cream where she had the splint after the fracture.
Client: The doctors didn't believe me, they thought nothing was broken. But I knew, and after ten days of uncertainty I asserted myself and made them carry out a CT! Luckily, I was true to myself, she says triumphantly. And she continues: After that I felt reassured, and it healed really quickly and well . . . Now both arms and hands feel relaxed.

The therapist asks the client to stand on the spot she had chosen for the shame. She immediately feels herself getting smaller and shrinking. She is reminded of many times when there was pain and the impulse to hide. Now she remembers the time of her teeth straightening. Between the ages of 7 and 14, she was picked on because of her teeth. To conceal her ugly teeth, she did not allow herself to laugh. She reports how the braces were tightened weekly, after which the pain was so strong for three days that she couldn't eat. So, she always ate a lot of chocolate before going to the dentist to survive the days of hunger.

The therapist invites her to stand on the spot of dignity again. Now the feeling of uprightness is even stronger. The client feels bigger.

Client: I was extremely strong and brave that I managed so well for seven years. The dentist kept praising me for it.

Therapist: Amazing, how strong you were, suffering these tortures week in and week out for seven long years and yet still continuing! Where in your body do you feel this strength?

Client: In my center, my spine and in the connection to the ground.

The therapist invites the client once more to stand on the spot of shame, and asks her to feel inside and notice her body sensations.

Client: I'm not so small anymore. And yes, it is remarkable how I kept going despite the terrible pain and having to starve for days. My mouth was all tense because I always had to keep my lips together, it was so exhausting. And my speech was also impaired.

Therapist: To keep going for so long was indeed a tour de force! Wow! That takes a lot of inner strength. This shame pertains to those others who shamed, offended, and belittled you – not to you.

The client, having been invited by the therapist to do so, switches back to her place of dignity, where she now feels even bigger, and also calm, centered, and grounded.

Therapist: Would you like to say something to the little one who feels so ashamed?

The client turns towards the "shame spot" and says: I understand that you felt ashamed. You were different, people noticed you. However, from my present adult perspective you have no reason to be ashamed. Rather, the others should be ashamed. You suffered and were so strong. And I appreciate your perseverance and your discipline. That was quite an achievement.

Therapist: Tell her that it will not last forever!
Client: It will not only pass but you will also have beautiful teeth and be able to laugh and to beam with joy!

The therapist asks the client to go back to the shame position once again and to feel what it feels like now.

Client: It was important to hear that it doesn't pertain to me, that I can actually be proud of my achievement and that it will pass. Now I feel good here as well.

To complete the process, the therapist invites the client to switch to the place of dignity and again, to absorb the sense of dignity and of being big into her body.

Client: Now I feel complete, quiet, and calm, dignified, like a swan. I can be as big as I am.

As just described, deep shame is not only an existential threat but also a state of collapse and immobility, which is why we worked with it while standing. In a standing position, it is easier for the client to feel her whole body and her balance, and it is much easier to start moving. The therapist is present, supporting, as necessary, in difficult moments with a soft touch at the upper arm (after having asked for permission) and inviting the client to pause once in a while and focus on her body. The therapist attends to the client's window of tolerance, making sure she does not stay in a state of shame for too long by inviting her to move or to switch to the position of dignity. She also differentiates: This shame does not pertain to you but to the others. You were shamed by the others! Finally, she invites the client to speak to the shamed part from the position of dignity, supporting her as much as needed – that is, as little as possible, but enough. In the example, the client had many years of experience in therapy and did not need much input from the therapist.

The process described is about "taking the shame to pieces" and deconstructing the frozen position of shame, allowing for something new to arise. In terms of Eugene Gendlin's (2003) Focusing approach, focusing on the body sensations entails a reorientation in the whole nervous system and in all parts of the brain, the organism literally realigning and organizing itself in a new way. There is a resolution that can be felt physically and a new insight, a whole new *experience*. Levine (2017) emphasizes that the critical change towards resolution comes from the body because solutions coming from the intellect are too swift and aim at avoiding the feelings of shame.

From an ego state perspective, the resource state of dignity is strengthened and anchored in the body. Then the shamed ego state is contacted, appreciated, and informed that the shame does not pertain to it. There is communication between the two parts: A strong ego state supports a weak one, eventually leading to integration and reorientation.

Compassion for the shame part allows the emotional and physical reactions to shift towards dignity and empowerment.

With all of the body-oriented interventions mentioned, it is helpful to *first only feel* the impulses to move, to notice them in a mindful way, *before* exploring micromovements and executing them in a titrated way. Sometimes it is not even necessary to actually do the movements. In people who are stuck in a frozen state, shifting position can speed up the change in such a way that the organism immediately switches into another state, which can be most helpful. There are many ideas, suggestions, and instructions how to do this. Maggie Phillips (2016) recommends *self-holding* or the *circle of strength* for self-regulation and strengthening of resources when there is shame. Both exercises are described in the last chapter.

O'Hanlon tells clients suffering from chronic shame: Maybe you will never get rid of this shame completely. But we can find out what triggers the shame to see how you can deal with these triggers (Buczynski, 2017, Video 7, Part 1).

Chronically Offended and Shamed

Michael Linden (2017), German neurologist and specialist for psychosomatic medicine, proposed a clinical picture he calls *posttraumatic resentment disorder*: One or more critical events affecting sensitive areas of our lives and perceived by the individual as being unjust, leading to deep mortification. If this mortification is not resolved, it entails resentment, aggression, and isolation. This disease pattern affects men and women of various ages equally, the basic mood ranging from dysphoric, aggressive to depressive. People see themselves as victims and react with resentment, anger, or hatred, when the relevant event is addressed. Consequently, they react with withdrawal, avoidance, spite, denial, and irreconcilability, accompanied by somatic complaints when there is no stable attachment and/or if the person experiences helplessness at the same time. The isolation primarily provides rescue and relief, but the bottom line is that it keeps the person in a feeling of being an outcast. Fear and pain, along with anger and a longing for revenge are reinforced. Resentment means abdicating our own development or, in the worst case, abdicating life.

In therapy, all these feelings can be expressed, heard, and understood. Depending on the client's needs the feelings can be strengthened, supported, or encouraged to communicate and cooperate. Ego states of *dignity* and *joy* that can help accompany people in this condition back into life need to be found. In this context, shame is seen as a "guardian of the inner shell," of the most precious core, the inner treasure. Once the different parts have been understood and strengthened, rehabilitated, or abolished, it is essential for the person affected to detach from having to resent something. If they can let go of bitter reproaches, they can open their heart and participate in life again (Bierbaum-Luttermann, 2011).

To let go of trauma, guilt, or emotional connections to an ex-partner, Emmerson's *Separation Sieve* can be used. This most useful metaphor for letting go works surprisingly well when used in the right moment. The instructions can be found in Chapter 8.

Bohne's *tapping technique* is equally helpful with clients suffering from self-reproaches or reproaches from others (2016). The client is invited to circle with their right hand on the heart area and, if possible, to repeat out loud, prompted by the therapist: Although I blame X for . . . I love and accept myself the way I am, leaving the responsibility for the other's behavior with X. The therapist joins in the movement, making circles with their hand. This "separation of responsibility" between the client and X through self-touch and the expression of sentences of self-acceptance usually creates a noticeable change of feelings towards relief and distance.

Moving from Guilt to Action

Real and Adopted Feelings of Guilt

As just described, there are healthy and unhealthy guilt feelings. You might also say that there are the *real guilt feelings* and those *imposed or transferred to us by others*. A prime example of the latter is guilt that has been passed on across generations. With real, healthy guilt feelings, the offense needs to be repaired in reality. If that is not possible, it can happen in therapy on the inner stage. This can be done with different procedures, one being Helen Watkins' *Door of Forgiveness* (Watkins & Watkins, 1997), another Emmerson's most useful *Separation Sieve* (2014). Please refer to Chapter 8 for instructions for both procedures.

A further possibility is the *tapping technique for self-reproaches* suggested by Bohne (2016). While circling with their right hand (similar to the instruction in the previous section) on the heart area (points of self-affirmation), clients repeat out loud several times, together with the therapist, the following sentence: Although I blame myself for . . . I love and accept myself the way I am. The therapist can find suitable words with the client: Although I blame myself for . . . I am okay the way I am, I will try to accept myself. The therapist explores with the client why they acted the way they did back then, why they did wrong. Usually, you find out that clients *could* not or, for certain reasons, did not *want* to act otherwise. Then the therapist invites the client to tap on the nail of their index finger and repeat the following sentence: And now I forgive myself with all my heart, because I realize that I could not/would not do otherwise. My word of honor! While saying this last sentence, clients hold up their right hand as if taking an oath. Most clients react with surprise or amusement, feeling great relief and a clear reduction of stressful feelings. Sometimes this needs to be repeated several times.

With *imposed guilt feelings* it is a bit more complicated. Here, an inner dialogue is required before clients can let go of their stressful emotions for good.

Disentangling Guilt Feelings through Inner Dialogue

According to Emmerson (2014), an ego state feeling guilty is "vaded with confusion." This state of confusion can be resolved, if the part can express its guilt feelings and enter a dialogue with the introject towards which it is feeling guilty. If clients distress themselves with self-reproaches, Emmerson suggests that an all-loving being such as God or Mother Earth be introduced, and that an empty chair for this all-loving being is used. Clients express their guilt feelings to the empty chair, to this being. Then they are invited to sit on the empty chair and to answer as God or Mother Earth. The almighty and all-loving being will forgive the client and also express it. If they do not, the therapist can remind them that they are not only almighty but also all-loving. Once clients have experienced forgiveness, they experience calm and relief.

If clients do not want to talk about the content of their guilt feelings because they feel ashamed, therapists might say: You don't have to tell me why you are feeling guilty. Then an empty chair is provided for the person towards whom the client feels guilty (or for the all-loving being). The client is guided: Please allow the person or being to sit on this chair and tell them quietly or out loud what you feel guilty for. Once clients have expressed their guilt feelings they are invited to sit on the chair (of the introject or the all-loving being) and to answer silently or out loud. Several exchanges may be needed until the inner dialogue can lead to clarity and resolution. Therapists keep instructing clients to pause and observe their reactions. They practice active listening by mirroring the essence of what the client is saying, the way they understand it intuitively.

How powerful and healing such an inner dialogue can be, can be seen in the following excerpt from the therapy with Marina, who was introduced earlier.

Marina, having been abused by her sports coach when she was six, already feels much better after we empowered the six-year-old and offered her corrective experiences. Her ego was strengthened and the connection to her resources are now intact.

Client: The anger is gone. The six-year-old is still feeling good. But that could change any moment. It would be nice to have even more safety, so that it can't change so quickly anymore.

When asked by the therapist what she needs now, Marina does not know, which is why the therapist suggests asking the subconscious. With Marina in a light trance, she accompanies her to her safe place (*strengthening resources*), and then asks Inner Knowledge what is needed so Marina can feel safer. Inner Knowledge replies that Marina should tell her parents. The client starts crying. The therapist suggests she might do this on the inner stage and asks the part that feels guilty towards the parents what she should call it.

Client: Bad Conscience.

Then the therapist asks Bad Conscience whether she needs company. She nods and would like to have Marina's boyfriend on her left. Now Bad Conscience, still crying, feels strong enough to tell her parents what happened with her coach and what she kept secret from them.

The therapist speaks directly to the parents' introjects: Have you heard what your daughter just said? What's that like for you?

Both parents are upset and hug their daughter, telling her how sorry they feel, exchanging love with her. The therapist emphasizes the loving connection between parents and "Bad Conscience" (*clarifying inner dialogue with the introjects*).

Therapist:	Bad Conscience, what's it like now?
Client as	I'm so happy and relieved!
Bad Conscience:	
Therapist:	Does the name Bad Conscience still fit? No? What may I call you now?
Client:	Relief.

After this intervention, grown-up Marina also feels relieved and free. She says she will think about telling her real parents about her coach's sexual assault. The therapist completes this third and last session with *resource strengthening* in a safe place.

Stabilization and complete healing of the trauma only occur after the guilt feelings of the client have been resolved through the inner dialogue with the parents' introjects.

Letting Go of Rumination

Besides guilt and shame, people affected by trauma are often also haunted by unpleasant rumination about experiences, the loss of a loved one or something else, making it difficult for them to concentrate on their work or to sleep well at night. This kind of rumination can involve feelings of guilt and shame, existential angst, or the conviction that the person or somebody else has done something wrong. Constant worries about another person, or feelings of uncertainty after contact with an important other has been broken off, can also be associated with rumination. Like guilt, shame, anger, blaming, or inconsolable grief, constant rumination prevents letting go of the past and advancing in life. Although the factors mentioned are quite different, the therapeutic interventions are similar, for, according to Emmerson (2014), rumination is related to a part overwhelmed *with confusion*. To let go, this state needs to express itself, to dialogue and clarify with the relevant introject on the inner stage. Emmerson suggests working with chairs to enable the client to communicate with the introjects (Changing Chairs Introject Action). *Working with chairs* underlines the clear distinction between client and introject. Incidentally, working with chairs is also suitable for the work with ego states in people with personality disorders or with a dissociative identity disorder.

Note

1 Unstable platform, which can trigger healing impulses. As the body seeks its balance, an outward orientation of attention automatically takes place, away from the intrusive events within.

References

Bierbaum-Luttermann, H. (2011): *Krank durch Kränkung und Beschämung.* (Workshop Teile-Therapie-Congress, 24–27 November 2011, Heidelberg, Germany).

Bohne, M. (2016): *Klopfen mit PEP. Prozess- und Embodimentfokussierte Psychologie in Therapie und Coaching.* Heidelberg: Carl Auer.

Buczynski, R. (2017): *A Way to Heal Trauma-Based Shame Using a 3-Dimensional Space.* In: B. van der Kolk & B. O'Hanlon (2017): *How to Work with Shame when it's Connected to Trauma.* The National Institute for the Clinical Application of Behavioral Medicine (Webinar).

Bull, N. (1962): *The Body and Its Mind: An Introduction to Attitude Psychology.* New York: Las Americas.

Emmerson, G. (2014): *Resource Therapy. The Complete Guide with Case Examples & Transcripts.* Victoria: Old Golden Point.

Erikson, E. H. (1950): *Childhood and Society.* New York: W.W. Norton & Co.

Gendlin, E. T. (2003): *Focusing. How to Get Direct Access to your Body's Knowledge.* Revised and updated 25th anniversary edition. E-Book. London: Random House.

Lanius, R. A. et al. (2002): Brain Activation During Script-driven Imagery-induced Dissociative Responses in PTSD. A Functional MRI Investigation. *Biological Psychiatry, 52,* 305–311.

Levine, P. (2017): *Shame and Pride.* (Seminar in Weggis, Switzerland (12–15 August 2017).

Linden M. (2017): *Verbitterung und Posttraumatische Verbitterungsstörung.* Göttingen: Hogrefe.

Marks, S. (2016): *Scham. Die tabuisierte Emotion.* (Patmos) 6. Aufl.

Phillips, M. (2016): *How to Heal Trauma and Pain Through the Body: Somatic Psychotherapy Level 3,* (Seminar in Zurich, 30 September–1 October 2016).

van der Kolk, B. (2017): *How to Work with Shame.* Video 7, Part 1. www.nicabm.com.

Watkins, J., & Watkins, H. (1997): *Ego States. Theory and Therapy.* W.W. Norton & Company.

Zanotta, S. (2013): *Das Monster zum Freund machen: Hypnosystemische Behandlung von Angst und Phobie.* Workshop. 7. Kindertagung Heidelberg. www.auditorium-netzwerk.de.

Chapter 7

Pain and Somatic Symptoms

Pain can result from physical injuries or impairments. However, unresolved trauma also leads to tenseness or freeze in the body due to posttraumatic stress, bringing about changes in organs and causing or intensifying pain. Chronic pain per se is traumatizing because it is overwhelming and triggers feelings of powerlessness. Emotional and physical pain are conducted through the same nerve tracts; hence it can be treated in the same way. To transform physical and emotional pain, the parasympathetic nervous system (ventral vagus) must be activated through *relaxation techniques*, such as hypnosis, meditation, massage, and yoga, all of which help reduce stress and promote the healing process. With a strong pain syndrome, medication in the right dose, applying heat or cold, trigger point injections, etc. are needed for a reliable pain relief. Moreover, it is important to *reduce negative emotional states* increasing the probability of pain triggers, and to build *resilience*. With chronic or strong pain, this often seems to be impossible. Activating resilience is even more difficult when freezing or dissociation paralyze the organism. To protect from pain, the freeze reaction releases opiates and endorphins in the organism. If it is not resolved and dissociation persists, resilience cannot be experienced. Resolving the traumatic tension allows for resilience, consolidation, and expansion, soothing the pain or even making it disappear (Phillips 2014, 2016).

Building Resilience

- Connecting with others
- Accepting that challenges are part of being alive
- Focusing daily on goals and dreams, taking the next step
- Doing anything (no matter how little), to confront the distress/misery, so as to come to terms with it
- Observing, how becoming active makes one feel better
- Seeking possibilities of self-discovery and empowerment
- Nourishing positive self-concepts

DOI: 10.4324/9781003460602-8

- Holding onto hope, finding inspiration
- Seeking help, if necessary
- Investing in self-care

Besides relaxation and stress reduction – the stress hormone cortisol can slow down the healing process and increase pain – enough *sleep* is important. Lack of sleep creates stress and exhaustion. A regular sleeping rhythm is essential to the healing process. To achieve this with sleeping disorders is at least as challenging as alleviating the pain. With long-standing symptoms and massive insomnia, it is often necessary to assist the process carefully with non-addictive medication, whilst at the same time teaching self-regulation and self-soothing techniques such as self-hypnosis and the activation and creation of images of rest. With sleeping disorders, careful psychoeducation, a new time management before sleeping, and the development of calming rituals are also necessary to prepare the organism for sleep (Phillips, 2016).

Furthermore, it is useful to *record* the pain precisely with pain charts. This leads to a differentiated perception of the occurrence of pain and to uncovering the trigger pattern or the pain trigger. This also incites clients to take charge, allowing them to become active and take distance from their experience of pain. Maggie Phillips suggests the following 10-step model for pain treatment (Phillips, 2007).

10-Step Model for the Treatment of Pain (Phillips, 2007)

1. Breathing techniques, to shift the pain and enhance positive feelings
2. Self-regulation through body awareness, tracking sensations
3. Reliable relaxing techniques: Feel the pleasure around pain
4. Change the pain image
5. Cultivate mindfulness and spirituality
6. Find your healing energy
7. Move away from pain, become active
8. Pendulate to disconnect pain from past trauma, to dissolve fight/flight/freeze reactions
9. Embrace the heart of your pain: Clearing emotional and physical pain
10. Build on success, get into the "yes" set

This process incorporates moving-pausing-perceiving-breathing-imagining and connecting the different nervous systems and brain areas.

Alleviating Pain and Somatic Symptoms with Ego State Therapy

In addition, Ego State therapy can support the healing of pain. Emmerson was able to show in a study that migraine is very often dominated by a state, and that the level of migraine correlates with depression or anger. The study features remarkable results: Using Ego State therapy, the frequency of migraine attacks could be reduced to a fifth of what they were (Emmerson & Farmer, 1996).

Emmerson distinguishes between more *psychosomatically* caused disorders like tension headaches, migraine, or asthma on the one hand, and symptoms which are largely *somatic*, such as physical injuries, organ disorders, or mental disorders largely caused genetically (for example, ADHD or bipolar disorders). He recommends different procedures for the two categories: If the pain is *psychosomatic*, the therapist tries to help the state responsible or even causing it. With *organically* caused pain, an appropriate resource part is asked for help. Often the symptom cause is unclear. Allergies, for example, can be of psychosomatic or organic origin. Careful medical examinations are therefore important. Pain that corresponds to certain situations or is associated with stress indicate a psychosomatic origin. If the pain occurs irregularly, independently of a situation, it can be both of organic and of psychosomatic nature.

If the origin cannot be determined, Emmerson recommends first applying the *psychosomatic* intervention. If, with this procedure, no state responsible for or associated with the symptom can be found, the intervention for organically caused pain is applied: A resource part that can help and take on the pain is identified.

Inversely, the therapist should never ask for a helping state when the problem is of a *psychosomatic* nature. This would cause a tug of war between the causative part and the part that was called for help, aggravating the symptoms (Emmerson, 2014).

Psychosomatic pain or symptoms are normally caused by a scared or neglected, rejected ego state, as seen in the next example. Sometimes, retro or conflicted parts can be responsible.

The 63-year-old client suffers from sometimes massive trigeminal pain occurring when she is too stressed and neglects self-care in order to adapt. Hypnosis, osteopathy, and medication have not brought the success she was hoping for. After a *conflict-free experience* in the first session in which she is able to set clear boundaries and in which she feels deeply touched, a *safe place* is established and *pendulation* happens in further therapy sessions. Spontaneously, the sentence pops up: I'm in charge, so she realizes that both states are present: Pain/powerlessness *and* resources/strength.

In the following sessions several small, frightened ego states show up, due to current crises and mortifications, which are strengthened, brought into the present, and connected with other strong parts.

In the fifth session the therapist asks about the part causing the pain. A crying baby appears, which the client can take onto her lap and soothe. The baby needs loving grandparents who can take care of her from now on and stay with her.

Client: The baby always needs to be held.

With the permission of the client, the therapist wraps a scarf around her shoulders, instructing her to hold her upper arms so she can also feel the corrective experience physically. Touching and holding her upper arms are good for her (*Containment*).

After this session the client has to take considerably less pain medication and can, over time, finally discontinue them altogether. She also touches and holds her upper arms at home over and over, thinking of the baby now being well taken care of and remaining safe with the grandparents. Holding her upper arms at home is also stabilizing and soothing. It is good and a relief for her. In the following sessions she reports that she is no longer so overwhelmed by the pain and that it only occurs occasionally.

Here, the pain symptoms are clearly reduced, nearly completely suspended, after the crying baby could have a corrective experience. The procedure is holistic, top-down and bottom-up, combining Ego State therapy with Somatic Experiencing®. Only later in the course of the therapy does it become apparent that the client was fed much too quickly and impatiently. Baby food was literally pressed into her mouth with the spoon.

References

Emmerson, G. J., & K. Farmer (1996): Ego State Therapy and Menstrual Migraine. *Australian Journal of Clinical Hypnotherapy and Hypnosis*, *17*: 7–15.

Emmerson, G. (2014): *Resource Therapy. The Complete Guide with Case Examples & Transcripts*. Victoria: Old Golden Point.

Phillips, M. (2016): *How to Heal Trauma and Pain Through the Body: Somatic Psychotherapy Level 3*, (Seminar in Zurich, 30 Sept.–1st Oct. 2016).

Phillips, M. (2014): *Somatic Experiencing for Psychotherapists who work with trauma &/or Ego State therapy, level 1* (Seminar in Zurich, 16–17 May 2014).

Phillips, M. (2007): *Reversing Chronic Pain: A 10-Point All-Natural Plan for Lasting Relief*. North Atlantic Books U.S.

Chapter 8

Pratical Applications in Therapy

A Therapy with a Somatic Focus

Early attachment ruptures, preverbal trauma, as well as complex traumatization are consistently challenging to psychotherapists, because the ego states and the psychophysiological processes involved are difficult to get at and influence. According to Porges' (1995) polyvagal theory, the system that is the most difficult to access and at the same time the most important in trauma healing is the dorsal-vagal circuit associated with the freeze or collapse reaction and dissociation. Many therapists are afraid of these shutdown reactions because the client's rupture of contact which comes up automatically triggers feelings of defense, anger, or helplessness in the therapist. Here, *coregulation* applies once again, besides principles such as psychoeducation and mindful accompaniment with somatic approaches and Ego State therapy. It is important that therapists keep taking time to regulate themselves in order to activate their inner observer and at the same time stay completely present. Having thus settled, they can then have a calming effect on the clients. This is not always possible, which is why s*upervision, intervision*, and s*elf-care* are indispensable for trauma therapists.

When clients are in a state of chronic sympathetic arousal, they need a counterpart who helps them tolerate and balance their feelings and sensations. Not only is it important to instruct clients on how to self-care with *grounding breathing exercises, mindfulness training*, and *self-regulation techniques*, practical *social support* in everyday life also plays a vital role. Luise Reddemann (2007) emphasizes how much of a priority "exterior safety" is for trauma healing.

The Somatic Experiencing® approach, with its *pendulation* according to Levine (2015, 2011, 2010, 1997) offers an extremely helpful and time-tested instrument both for freezing and hyperarousal. Clients are invited to pendulate back and forth between active (adrenal-vagal) and passive (dorsal-vagal) systems and between traumatic and resilient states. Through this activation of the natural pendulation rhythm of the autonomic nervous system, clients' inherent power of self-healing is activated, having a psycho-physiologically regulating and stabilizing effect. By combining this with Ego State therapy, young preverbal states that are often stuck in the freeze reaction at the time of the traumatic event because of their poorly

DOI: 10.4324/9781003460602-9

developed coping strategies, can also be contacted. Sensations typical for these preverbal states, such as cold, freezing, numbness, emptiness, and total helplessness are explored and the somatic preverbal parts involved located. With breathing techniques and mindful awareness of the sensory-motor experience, these trauma-associated reactions can be resolved. In *Somatic Ego State Therapy*, the body remains the most important vessel for resonance, showing in a reliable and direct way whether an intervention is right in that specific moment – both in the client and the therapist. For many therapists it is a relief that they do not always have to know the next step and can find out what direction to take together with the client by exploring body sensations. Clients can be invited to "ask the body" whether something is good or not, the (body's) response being quick and clear. The advantage of body work is also that there are no cultural or linguistic barriers to overcome. Moreover, the somatic focus in Ego State therapy is extremely effective with preverbal trauma, somatic symptoms, and difficulties with self-regulation. By switching from a passive freeze or depressive collapse to active self-assertion or flight, preverbal traumata can be resolved. It is more effective to have clients act out defense strategies and healthy self-assertion, thus experiencing them physically, than it is to use talk as the sole means of expression.

Holistic: Top-down and Bottom-up

The different possibilities of self-regulation have already been addressed and are summarized in Table 8.1. Methods operating through the prefrontal cortex, emphasizing cognition as well as attentional control or mindful body awareness, are called top-down methods. They are used to expand body awareness and to establish a safe meta-position supposed to register processes happening and supporting them through the ability to observe, the focus being on meaning and understanding. In addition, bottom-up approaches build on primarily exploring the interaction between sensation and movement. With the bottom-up focus, clients direct their attention to sensory-motor experiences and observe their interplay with feelings and thoughts, thus learning to be aware of their reactions to old and new somatic patterns and how they change. Thus, individuals can learn how their thoughts and

Table 8.1 Methods to regulate top-down- and bottom-up processes

Top-down	Bottom-up
Hypnosis	Breathing techniques
Ego State therapy	Tapping techniques, self-touch
Psychoeducation	Focusing, Somatic Experiencing® (Pendulation)
Mindfulness	Movement
Meditation	Changing posture/facial expression
Stories	Creative expression
Affirmations	Role play, play, dance

emotions affect their bodies, and how physical experiences, thoughts, and beliefs influence their emotions.

This holistic multimodal procedure embodies *Somatic Ego State Therapy*, which, being a combination of hypnosis, Ego State therapy, and a somatic focus, facilitates access to unconscious memories in the implicit memory and the resolution of early childhood trauma. Besides using tools from Focusing and Somatic Experiencing® therapy, therapists can work directly with the traumatized, non-integrated parts with Ego State therapy interventions, which make this contribution so valuable.

Safety with Clear Structures

As mentioned, clear structures are central to establishing a safe context. This includes a carefully settled therapeutic contract and continuity in and between sessions. Phillips (2016) suggests dividing the session into three parts: The first, to "meet" the clients where they are at; the second to work on the trauma; and the last to summarize and learn exercises. It is always useful to take time at the start and at the close of each session to clarify the presence of the client's resources – and not just in trauma therapy. This stabilizes and connects clients with their strong personality parts. Later in therapy, they will be better protected from being overwhelmed if they can feel safe before and after the confrontation with their difficult issues and leave the office in a stable state. Paulsen (2009) calls this principle the "resource sandwich."

In the first third of the session therapists might ask:

"What is important for you today? What would you wish for today? How have you been since the last time?"

Continuity and coherence can also be reinforced, if the therapist summarizes briefly the most important interventions, topics, and ego state processes of the last session and asks the client how these ego states are doing now. This not only allows for a reality check by inquiring about coping on a day-to-day basis – that is, do the therapeutic steps translate into daily life? – it also helps to find out whether additional stabilizing interventions for individual ego states or the entire personality are necessary after the last session. Along the lines of the therapy section with the 40-year-old client (Chapters 2 and 4), therapists are well advised to let clients decide when the time is ripe to work through the issue. Not all clients are able to sense, let alone communicate, that they need pauses and nourishment for the entire personality. Moreover, most psychotherapists tend to want to move forward too quickly. This is why it is important to take enough time at the beginning of the session to meet clients where they are and to explore carefully together with them what exactly they need. Regarding further therapeutic steps, therapists can take notes, so they can get back to them in a later session.

Often clients cannot remember the topics of the last session, which surprises or disturbs them. This can be used as a resource by reframing it:

> "Your unconscious always means well and knows exactly which memories are important to your healing. We do not always need to know everything with our intellect, for there is great wisdom in our organism. Sometimes problems can even be resolved more easily if you just let the unconscious processes happen. What is it like for you now that I tell you this?"

For the final third of the session, you can suggest exercises for clients to use in daily life. Many clients appreciate recording these exercises on their mobiles so that they can listen to them between sessions. Also, you can explore together whether and how the exercises tested in the session can be integrated into everyday life. With desperate, unstable clients it is often difficult to complete the session, because often just before the end of the session something urgent pops up. Clarity is helpful here too . . .

> "We now have five minutes left, then the session will be over. Is there something that is important for you now? What do you need to complete this session in a good way? Or: When this session ends in a few minutes where do you want to be? How do you want to feel when you walk through that door?"

Occasionally, needy traumatized ego states associated with a high arousal of the client, show up with some urgency, whereupon the therapist might say to the client:

> "I can see that there are other younger parts that are still desperate or stuck in the past. Do you agree that we promise all those parts to take care of them in a later session . . . because we now only have five minutes left? However, these younger ego states deserve to be taken care of appropriately and to be given the time they need. Is there a place where they would be safe until we can do that so that they do not have to suffer anymore? Somewhere, where all suffering parts would be on holiday and safe, as it were? I don't know where that could be, maybe on an island, in a cave, or in a garden? Only you know what exactly they need!"

With the support of the therapist the client then brings all the suffering ego states to a place where they are safe and protected and can settle until it is time for their integration. The client promises them that from now on they will take care of them. The therapist also makes a note and picks it up at a later date. Yet often, not all these ego states need to be nourished individually and retrospectively, rather a few of them can be integrated vicariously. This intervention of "bringing states collectively to a safe place" when many needy ego states with high urgency all of sudden pop up has a rather rapid calming effect, gives the clients a level of control, and allows therapists to complete the session on time.

Self-regulation – An Important Resource at the Beginning of the Therapy

It is worthwhile trying out different self-regulation and grounding methods with the client so you can find out together what is most helpful.

Many people learned in childhood, in the presence of trauma, that it isn't safe to experience emotions, or to be present in their bodies, aware of body sensation. Cutting those feelings and sensations off was a survival strategy during times of trauma, abuse or neglect. Highly dissociative clients especially need to learn grounding procedures as an early step to intervene in their chronic sense of being unreal, empty or outside of themselves.

(Paulsen, 2009, p. 103)

Grounding Exercises

With grounding exercises, clients can learn to focus on existing resources, to orient in the present or, if they are afraid of their inner experiences, to direct their attention to something soothing in their immediate environment.

- Finding a safe, pleasant, or strong place in the body
- Connecting with inner resources (internal strength, resourceful ego states, place of wellbeing, safe place)
- Finding a spot, a color, an object in the environment that is good and soothing when looking at it
- Standing up, moving
- Pressing one's heels into the ground
- Feeling the materials of the furniture or other objects in the environment
- Naming five things and their color in the immediate environment
- Smelling a fragrance (lavender, sage, orange blossom)
- Tasting salt
- Petting an animal
- Grounding breathing exercises (outlined in the next sections)

Distancing Techniques

With people suffering from dissociation or flashbacks, the following distancing techniques can be important, in addition to grounding exercises:

- Establishing an "inner observer" state
- Taking a bird's eye view
- Screen technique (Reddemann, 2007)
- Counter images, developing counter thoughts as an antidote to the trauma
- Pendulating to the resource
- Standing up, moving
- Orienting to the present, towards the outside

Breathe First!

A good method of entry into self-regulation is mindful breathing. When we are breathing mindfully, directing our attention to our breathing, awareness and body are being connected to each other, we are immediately activating the parasympathetic nervous system. Mindful breathing can change the frequency of the brain waves, from beta to alpha waves. Victims of unresolved trauma tend to breathe with tension as part of their freeze reaction. The simple technique of paying attention to diaphragmatic respiration is generally very helpful, the aim being primarily to be aware of the breathing rather than wanting a change. Presented in the right way, this is possible with any client. You can even "sell" breathing techniques to adolescents, for example, as a way of improving their performance in their favorite athletic or school activity.

The easiest breathing exercise, which immediately activates the ventral vagus, was suggested by Levine, Porges, and Phillips (2015, pp. 35–36):

"Inhale briefly through your nose, then exhale slowly and as long as possible through your mouth."
"You can try to gradually extend the phases of exhale by counting."

And here's a short, consolidating exercise recommended by Maggie Phillips (2014):

"Think of a resource, a strength, a situation, in which you felt safe and strong. Find the associated energy in your body. On the inhale, focus on this energy, breathing into this energy, on the exhale, think 'now' or 'letting go' or 'enjoying' and let anything unpleasant or disturbing go. Repeat! How does that feel? If you can feel this energy of strength or safety or some kind of well-being clearly, you can amplify it by tapping on the back of your hand, tapping in between the metacarpal of the little and of the ring finger with three or four fingers, thus amplifying and anchoring this energy."

Such simple exercises lead to a quicker symptom reduction, particularly with pain or high arousal, which is especially important at the beginning of therapy. You help clients to experience themselves as being self-effective and to gain more control over themselves and the hope for healing of trauma, fear, or depression.

Connecting Breathing with Imagination

Clients can also be instructed to combine their breathing with images.

"Imagine your body being surrounded by a healing energy field, a healing color, a healing light . . . healing sounds or just a healing presence. On the inhale, imagine that you let this light, this sound, this healing presence stream into your belly and chest and then everywhere into your body. On the exhale, imagine your body letting go of anything unpleasant, tension, discomfort, pain, stress. Repeat this respiratory cycle four or five times. On the inhale, the healing energy flows into the body; on the exhale, anything unpleasant flows out. On the inhale, the energy flows into every fiber, every cell of your body; on the exhale it flows out again. When it is time to end this little exercise, focus your attention again on your surroundings."

Simple, Grounding Breathing Exercises

There are also very simple breathing exercises where you put your hand on the diaphragm and observe how something moves out or lifts when inhaling and returns to the initial position when exhaling.

Grounding breathing exercises:

"Push the pads of your feet softly into your shoes or on the floor when inhaling and let go when you are exhaling. Repeat two or three times. How's that? What do you notice?"

Or:

> "When inhaling, gently press the palm of your hands onto your thighs while pressing your pads, and let go when exhaling. Repeat two or three times. How's that?"

Or:

> "Make a fist and clench it while inhaling, let it go when exhaling."

Or:

> "Press your hands against each other when inhaling, let them go when exhaling."

Mindful Breathing (Phillips, 2008)

> "Explore the here and now: What do you see in your mind's eye? What do you feel? What are you thinking? What images do you have? Name them to yourself.
>
> Accept with love and compassion for yourself that this is your experience in this moment. With the next inhale, stop everything you are presently mindfully aware of with your breath, then let it all go with your exhale.
>
> With the next inhale, step into a new here and now. Be open to what you meet in this new moment. Name everything you are mindfully aware of. Stop that as well with your breath and then let it go with your exhale.
>
> Repeat this cycle if needed."

Other breathing techniques, like the circular breathing, can be found in Maggie Phillips' book *Reversing Chronic Pain* (Phillips, 2007), where she describes the following variations of mindful breathing:

> **Diaphragmatic respiration**: Put both hands on the diaphragm area. On the inhale, press your feet against the floor and on the exhale let go again.
>
> **Circular breathing** supports the pendulation rhythm of the nervous system and is therefore helpful for flight, fight, or freeze reactions. It is mainly

used with trauma and nerve pain. Imagine that your breath flows up one side of your body as you inhale and goes down the other side of your body as you exhale. It is usually more effective to link breathing in with the less painful side . . . and breathing out with the more painful side (p. 22).

3-point-respiration increases safety, control, presence, leading "from worry to wonder." *Inhale – hold – exhale*: It is safe, I can feel how the chair, the universe is holding me. I'm curious what my body will do with this extra energy that I am giving it when I stop worrying and start wondering instead.

For back pain: On the inhale, observe how more space is created between the ribs and the vertebrae and the spine lengthens . . . exhale and let go. Yes, inhaling fully makes for more space between the vertebrae. And, you can imagine how the spine gets longer, allowing for more oxygen and blood to flow into it.

These breathing exercises should be done several times a day for one minute. To center and emotionally stabilize yourself, it is helpful to connect the conscious with the unconscious (Phillips, 2008).

Self-regulation through Over-energy Correction

Process and Embodiment Focused Psychology (PEP) by Michael Bohne offers the following simple and very effective exercise, allowing clients to soothe themselves and gain distance from their inner restlessness or feeling of stress quite quickly, which, in turn, reinforces self-efficacy in the regulation of emotions.

The Over-energy Correction

The following figure illustrates this simple exercise, which can bring about energetic balance. Sitting with crossed hands and feet on a chair, you slightly touch your palate with the tip of your tongue while inhaling, letting go when exhaling.

While sitting on a chair, stretch both legs, placing the left ankle over the right one, so that the ankles are on top of each other.

Extend both arms forward and put the left wrist over the right one, palms against each other, fingers interlaced.

Rotate the crossed wrists upward so they come to rest on your chest.

Close your eyes. On the inhale, press the tip of your tongue against your palate. On the exhale, let go of the palate with your tongue. Repeat this exercise three or four times or until you feel a shift towards more balance, calm, or wellbeing.

Variation:

For this exercise to be effective, the posture must feel unfamiliar, meaning you can do it the other way round: The right leg over the left leg, the right wrist over the left wrist.

Effect of the exercise:

- Brings more attention, calm, and concentration
- Supports being emotionally centered
- Improves physical coordination and balance
- Brings more wellbeing, boosts ability to set boundaries

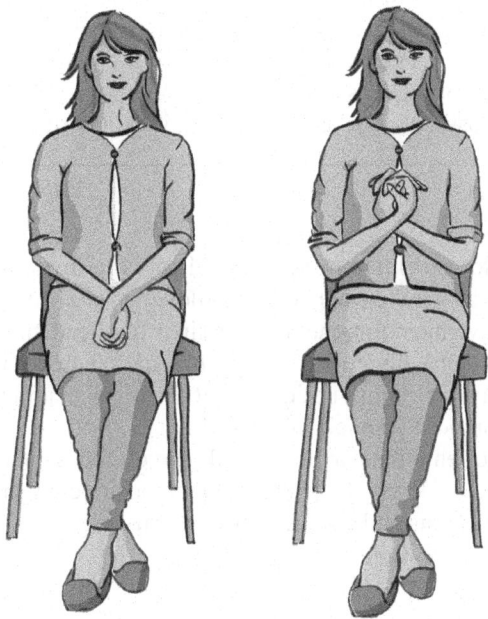

Figure 8.1 Over-energy correction

The therapist can accompany the crossing of the limbs with the following words:

"With this crossing, the unfamiliar is what is important . . . through the unfamiliar crossing of arms and legs many areas of the brain are activated . . ., animating them to link and cooperate . . ., which opens you up for new experiences. . . .

On the inhale through the nose: Touch your palate with your tongue behind the upper incisors, letting go on the exhale . . . With this, even more brain areas are activated, especially those in the brainstem regulating our autonomic involuntary body processes . . .

This is why touching with the tongue on the inhale and letting go on the exhale is so important . . . You can support this process of energy balance, of self-regulation . . . making it more pleasant . . . by visualizing an image of balance . . .

I don't know what that is for you . . . maybe a scale with its trays in balance . . . a picture or an experience of yourself being in balance . . . or a picture from nature . . ., maybe the sea, waves coming and going . . . or something else . . .

Allow your breath to flow naturally . . ., while your tongue touches the upper palate on the inhale . . ., letting go on the exhale . . . and observe what that is like for you . . . Only you know when it is enough, and your body can slowly move out of this position . . ."

Afterwards, ask: "How was that? What did you notice?"

Self-touch can also contribute to settling. Clients are invited to cross their arms and to put their hands on their upper arms, allowing for a feeling of being held. An alternative is to have them put one hand on their forehead, the other on their heart or both hands on their belly above the diaphragm. Wherever their hands come to rest, they are always invited to notice how it feels: "Is that pleasant? Unpleasant? How is it when you hold yourself like that?"

The following orientation exercise, in which you focus on a resource in the surroundings first, is also strengthening and has a positive effect on self-regulation. Noticing body sensations and feeling them helps us connect to inner resources and creates additional connections.

Orientation Exercise

Position yourself comfortably and find a resource in your surroundings that you like looking at. Notice how that affects your inner state of being and connect with the resulting body sensation.

Now connect with a familiar resource and the corresponding body sensation. Pendulate back and forth between the two resources/body sensations.

Now engage even more deeply in your body sensations until you have the feeling that the experience is complete.

Learning to Name Sensations

The question – How does it feel in your body? – does not always allow for a quick answer. Many clients first have to learn to name their sensations so they can actually feel the body sensations of strength and safety and make a connection to their body. As explained earlier, the development of the brain is shaped by sensations, which is why positive joyful experiences are essential for children and adolescents. The same applies to unstable, desperate, low-spirited, and frightened or panicking people. Besides (re)focusing their attention on small, beneficial everyday experiences, in line with Reddemann's joy journal (Reddemann, 2007), and practicing pendulation to the counter thought, clients must learn the *language of sensations*.

When clients have practiced in therapy naming their body sensations and to feel what they need, it often translates into daily life where needs are more clearly noticed and expressed.

Therapists can offer their clients a multiple choice of words to help them describe their sensations.

While the clients feel into their sensations, mindfully accompanied and titrated by the therapist, they move through one cycle of soft activation and relaxation of the nervous system, spontaneously integrating parts of their consciousness, mobilizing sensory-motor energies, and restoring, developing, and organizing physiological and affective states. Clients get centered, finding their strength, physical balance, and an appropriate muscle tone, thus returning to the present. During the process of sensing, they are invited to keep pausing, notice minimal changes, and thus perceive subtle differences.

Table 8.2 Multiple choice of body sensations

light – heavy	soft – hard
stabbing – tingly	tense – easy
flowing – blocked	cool – warm
cold – hot	bright – dark
strained – open	jittery – quiet
full of energy – tired	weak – strong
grounded – beside oneself	shaky – stable
wide – tight	restless – still
slow – fast	numb – hypersensitive
tingling – tickly	blurred – clear
opening – burning	airy – stuck
rising – sinking	humming – quiet

The goal of feeling mindfully and carefully into what they are sensing, and naming their body sensations, is the activation of the brainstem as the seat of autonomic survival reactions. The awareness of physical sensations is increased, slowing down physiological processes in the nervous system so that corrective experiences on all levels are possible.

The language of the therapist should be inviting and encouraging, slow, soft, and not hypnotic. Therapists offer suggestions, in accordance with the images surfacing in them, repeating and thus confirming the client's statements. They support the expansion and the connection with resources or the pendulation to empowering feelings, so that clients do not get stuck in unpleasant sensations for too long. Helpful formulations accompanying and supporting the process of perception include:

What do you notice/feel right now?

What is happening now?

Where (in your body) do you feel that?

Are you curious to find out . . .?

Do you agree to stay with this sensation for a moment? (Only for 15 seconds?)

Take a moment to feel and observe what that is like.

What would it feel like if you stayed with this feeling for a while?

The more you learn to trust your body . . .

How would you describe that? – I know that that is difficult, but it is so important!

Could you say more about that?

Tell me what that feels like. If it were an object, what would it be? A stone, a ball, a fist . . .? (Suggestions according to the images popping up spontaneously in the therapist)

Exactly. You feel this tingling in your right foot. (*Confirmative repetition*)

Observe what happens next. What is happening, while you stay with it?

When it (the unpleasant) gets more intense, find a place in your body that is not so . . . (i.e., tense)! Or: Direct your attention to your feet or the support of the chair you are sitting on. Or: See if you notice something in your environment here that gives you safety, lets you settle, no matter what it is.

You feel the lightness in your hands. Can you feel the lightness elsewhere in your body? (*Expanding*)

Good. And while you are feeling this strength in your legs, what does that remind you of? (*Connecting with other resources, possibly also in the body*)

Some clients may experience parts of their body as irritating or unpleasant (i.e., tense, painful), at which point the therapist can invite them to put their hand on that area and feel whether that makes a difference. As a next step, they can ask the client to "breathe into" this area a few times to explore the body sensations there. Often this not only leads to clients calming down and the symptoms being reduced, but also to resources and ideas for solutions arising spontaneously. Getting to know and reinforcing body resources stabilizes and increases the feeling of safety and therefore of resiliency.

Safe Place in the Body (Phillips, 2016)

> Where in your body is it somewhat more pleasant right now? If clients do not find anything: Take your time. You have all the time you need, just to notice where in your body it feels a bit calmer or warmer or stronger or just more pleasant. That might/could be in your belly or in your feet or back, in your hands? . . .
>
> The therapist allows the client to explore and name their sensations. Maybe you feel like putting your hand on that spot? Does it make a difference? Is it more pleasant, less pleasant? Again, clients describe their sensations. And now I'd like to invite you to breathe into that area . . . How's that?
>
> The client then describe their experience. "Is it a place where the entire person can rest? Imagine you're a cat, a dog, that can rest in this place with a feeling of security!"

Focusing – Mindful Experience in the Here and Now

Focusing not only means directing one's attention to one's body, it is also an attitude towards oneself: Being in contact with oneself, with all parts, in an unintentional and benevolent way. Focusing signifies taking time for mindful experiencing of what one is feeling and sensing, yet without knowing what it is or what it means. By pausing for a moment, giving attention and space, meaning and healing steps develop. It is about finding the "felt sense" and mindfully staying with it, which normally leads to relief and a solution. The "felt sense" is a holistic experience, is always new, in the here and now. It can only be felt if you give it the possibility to unfold (Gendlin, 2003).

Shifting Awareness/Pendulation

The above mentioned pendulation between tense and relaxed body areas helps reach an emotional-physical balance and supports mindful anchoring in the present.

Shifting Awareness (Levine, 2008; Maggie Phillips, 2016, 2014)

> 1. Explore the pain or symptom with the client.
> 2. Let clients assess the intensity of the problem on a scale of 1 to 10.

3. Explore the symptoms in the body and let the client describe the associated sensations or pain.
4. Ask about the place in the body that is furthest away from the symptom or feels like the opposite. (Where do you feel the opposite?)
5. Guide the client's focus back and forth, always giving them time to explore. Support them through your questions to stay with their body sensations and keep their focus. Take more time for the "pleasant" body area so that this sense is reinforced.
6. Let clients scale the intensity of the problem again (normally it clearly decreases; if that is not the case, go back to point 4 or give the client more time).
7. Now let clients also feel their breath to support the whole process: Focus on the positive or neutral body area when inhaling, bring attention to the symptom or the pain when exhaling. If this increases the unpleasant sensations, which is rather uncommon, the opposite procedure is advised: Inhale through the area of symptom and exhale through the pleasant area. Repeat throughout two or three respiratory cycles.
8. It is important to pause in order to explore the body sensations during the process: What do you notice? What do you feel?
9. Take some time to test it! Do you feel like continuing for a little while longer?
10. If clients want to end the exercise, you have them scale the intensity of the undesired experience again. Usually there is a marked improvement: You see, you alone have caused that. You can contribute to the relief!
11. Finally, clients may be invited to practice this it at home.

You can also pendulate/shift between two resourceful body areas to reinforce and connect them. Sometimes just shifting attention between two unpleasant areas can resolve trauma or pain without having to know its exact context or content.

The following instructions show how pendulation on the somatic level can resolve an inner conflict.

Quick Resolution of an Inner Conflict when One Part Resists Healing (according to Phillips, 2008)

Ask for a part of the self that wants to heal the pain (the part that insists on seeking help, wants to try something new, presses for psychotherapy, etc.).

Together with the client, find out where in the body this part lives. Explore this area by inquiring about sensations associated with it and intensify these with breathing techniques.

Then contact the ego state that is blocking the healing process/treatment. Together with the client, find out where in the body this part lives, mindfully noticing it and naming the sensations associated with it.

Invite the two parts to cooperate. If the body answer is "yes," you can instruct the client to pendulate between the two parts to gradually connect them. This connection can also be supported with the breath or imagination.

The Five-Minute Heart Intervention (based on Phillips, 2016)

1. Recognizing the emotional stress: Notice all unpleasant and energy robbing feelings or thoughts. These can be feelings of pressure or tension or feelings of powerlessness, tension, worry, guilt, reproach, upset, frustration, or fear . . .
2. Find the opposite feeling, for example: Ease, forgiveness, compassion, or appreciation, acceptance . . .
3. Where and when in your daily life can you access this opposite feeling? – Think of an everyday situation in which you have experienced this feeling.
4. Slowly and easily breathe the energy associated with the desired attitude or feeling in through your heart area and absorb the feeling. Take the time to anchor the feeling with the help of your breath.
5. This exercise helps your heart, your heart coherence, to change the reaction to stress and focus less on the emotional stress in favor of pleasant, soothing sensations and feelings.
6. You can also expand this exercise through the connection with other resources.

Changing Posture

Think of an irritating emotional state and explore the associated body sensations, thoughts, images, memories.

Let your body find a posture that embodies this state. Feel into it. How is that?

Without thinking about it: Now let your body take the opposite posture, allowing your body to take the lead.

Notice all the sensations, thoughts, and images that pertain to this posture.

Now let your body find a posture in between, a posture that is "just right."

Restoring Boundaries

Experiences of violated boundaries have to be recognized and named as such and acknowledged by the therapist. As in the work with the trauma vortex, it is important to remain "at the edge" of the unpleasant experience instead of getting lost in it. Therefore, therapists first explore where the boundaries are still intact and where it still feels safe for the client, proceeding gently, minding every little sign of activation of the client. If clients start bracing, protecting, or stiffening by minimally changing their posture, this is apparent in discreet changes of muscular tension around the eyes, the facial expression, posture, or breathing. Therapists immediately react by pausing and naming what they observe, and not forcing clients to take steps beyond this boundary. On the contrary, they move back to the counter vortex, back into the zone with intact boundaries that is safe for the client. Before approaching the "danger zone" gently and with minimal steps, therapists secure the client's consent. At the same time, therapists should consider the angle, distance, and direction of their position to the clients with whom they are sitting, exploring with the clients, what place in the room is best and safest for them.

Repairing Boundaries

- Clients choose a rope and lay out their "felt" personal boundary or they choose a color chalk and draw their boundary on the floor.
- As a support, symbols for resources or resource states can be put in this circle, "their territory."
- Therapists *gently* test this territorial boundary by moving in slow motion towards the side of the rope felt to be safe by the client, looking out for minimal body signals and immediately stopping when noticing the slightest "bracing." Usually, clients only notice then that they have laid out their boundary much too close. The boundary is continuously being adapted (normally expanded).
- Once the boundary has been established with the rope or the chalk, the client can be invited to try out stop signals, using their voice by saying (ever more loudly and clearly), Stop! Or No! The client can use gestures, for example, thrusting their palms outward in a protective and delimiting way. All the while, therapists give feedback and encourage a healthy delimitation and self-assertion until it is convincing and clear.
- The exercise is repeated until clients feel safe and protected.

Establishing New Boundaries

Once the boundary has been firmly established, the next step is to explore the perception of three-dimensional space carefully in a later session. Therapists move slowly along the rope, starting at the point where client feels safe and well, the client remaining in the center. At the smallest activation of the client, the therapist asks about their sensations. If the activation does not diminish, the therapist moves back to the safe zone until the client is ready again and gives the therapist permission to move back into the zone felt to be dangerous. Through this gentle pendulating procedure the activation settles gradually and new boundaries are established and consolidated.

Working in a Standing Position with Shame or Powerlessness

First, the therapist helps the client to take a posture of dignity, pride, or joy in a spot chosen by the client. Then, therapist and client collect and deepen together the sensations, images, thoughts, feelings, and movements according to the SIBAM model described in Chapter 2.

Think of a time when you felt proud or had a feeling of dignity and choose your posture accordingly. Let us explore the sensations that come with it. What does it feel like from head to toe?

The therapist accompanies this with understanding listening, joining in the posture, exploring as many details as possible so the state of dignity or joy can arise.

Subsequently, the client is encouraged to think of the shame and to find a suitable place and posture for the shame. It is advisable to choose another place in the room for this.

Stand a little bit more to the side. Now that you are standing on this spot, think of a moment when you felt shame – a shame that does not really belong to you but comes from outside. Can you feel how this sensation affects your body?

Usually, the terrible feeling now arises of shrinking, getting very small, or falling into powerlessness and helplessness, often accompanied by dizziness or nausea. A client must have enough time to feel the effects on their body but should also not stay in this state for too long so as not to be overwhelmed. You only explore until clients can sense the feelings clearly, and then immediately invite them to return to the place of dignity.

If it feels right, the therapist can speak directly to the powerless ego state and tell it that the past is over and that this shame does not belong to this state.

Back at the place of dignity, the therapist asks: How is it now? The therapist makes sure that there is eye contact. Do you feel the contact? How is that?

Now I'd like to ask you to return to the place of shame . . . how is it now?

Now the therapist lets the client pendulate between the two positions – or the two states – back and forth until the client experiences more flexibility, reflected immediately in their posture and movements. With the switching back and forth, the feeling of shame diminishes while the resource state becomes more dominant.

As an alternative, the therapist can ask the client when they are standing at the place of dignity what they would say to the part of them that is ashamed: Assuming the shame part is standing there, what would you like to tell it? . . . and what else?

Self-hug (Phillips, 2015)

One hand is resting on the forehead, the other on the chest: Calmly breathe in and out for a few minutes.

In a next step you put one hand on the forehead, while the other one is resting on the back of the head continuing to breathe calmly.

Now one hand rests on the chest, the other on the belly, also breathing quietly for a few minutes.

Then you can explore: Who feels held? Is it an ego state, and if so, what does it need?

Stabilizing and Strengthening through Ego State Therapy

Ego State therapy is an excellent way to help clients strengthen self-worth and connect to resources. This is not only constructive and builds trust at the beginning of the therapy but is also important later on. As seen in Chapter 2, humans automatically seek safety. This is not only about connecting with strong resourceful ego states and reintegrating traumatized parts through corrective experiences, but also the strengthening of the entire personality, especially in people with a fragmented psyche suffering from dissociative phenomena (Frederick & Phillips, 1995). If you only work with individual ego states you risk that the personality parts drift apart even more, which has a destabilizing effect. With the procedure described the entire personality is strengthened, because, for one thing, clients keep control and decide for themselves what the next step is and choose their own pace. People who have experienced a great deal of powerlessness need to stay in control in order to engage in therapy. Therapists can support this need with these types of statements:

"It is important to me that you always stay in control and keep control. *You* decide what is important for you in a session, and *you* determine how fast we proceed. I will always inform you about the steps and ask for your permission. I will ask you whether you are ready to take the next step. It is totally okay if there is something you do not want. Only you know and feel what is good for you. Should I forget this at some point, please remind me."

The therapist does not know in advance what the client needs exactly but rather tries to understand precisely, directing as little as possible, but also insisting until, for example, younger parts are fully rescued or safe places are completely safe.

Besides the control, safety plays an important role for the strengthening of the entire personality, the focus being on the outside safety in real life first: Are there current threats such as violence, abuse, other danger? Clients can obtain inner safety through corrective experiences on one hand, but also through *interventions strengthening the entire personality*, such as conflict-free experiences or inner strength, the safe place, inner wisdom, the inner healer, activating interventions.

Strengthening the Entire Personality

Being engaged with numerous inner parts can easily lead to confusion, losing track of the fact that Ego State therapy is, after all, about connection and integration, and strengthening the *entire* personality. The hypno-analytical concept of an "indestructible inner core" is not shared by all ego state schools, but all acknowledge a state of spiritual nature inherent to humans where they "rise above themselves," always a deeply touching experience. In Ego State therapy, techniques such as "inner strength," "inner wisdom," and "inner healer" can lead to this core self. Maggie Phillips calls this indestructible core *the Strong Self*; Emmerson speaks of the *Higher Self*, but says that you can only rarely activate this state of deep inner peace. By consolidating the strong self, stress hormones are reduced, the connection with the unconscious resources is strengthened, and more energy is available for healing.

"Conflict-free imagination" as offered by Phillips and Frederick (2010) is a very helpful intervention, often used early in therapy, and suitable for nearly all clients because it is based on *experiences* in reality. This is why we use the expression of *conflict-free experience*. It is self-invigorating and useful with clients who have a hard time with imagining or hypno-therapeutic concepts, because it ties in with experiences of daily life. Strengthening the entire personality has a stabilizing effect and promotes self-confidence and can also be obtained through the connection and cooperation of strong ego states, that is, through the *inner team*.

With these ego state concepts of strengthening the personality, the client's ability for imagination is improved, which is an important prerequisite for resilience.

We have seen that imagining an act engages the same motor and sensory programs that are involved in doing it . . . Everything your 'immaterial' mind imagines leaves material traces. Each thought alters the physical state of your brain synapses at a microscopic level. Each time you imagine moving your fingers across the keys to play the piano, you alter the tendrils in your living brain . . .

(Doidge, 2008, p. 505)

Conflict-free Experience

This section outlines the procedure for creating a conflict-free experience, along the lines of the conflict-free zone of Phillips and Frederick (2010).

1. Invite clients to think of a certain stressor, pain, or symptom.
2. Let them envision a conflict-free experience.
3. Help the client to build up an imagined experience as conflict-free. Reinforce it by exploring body sensations, images, thoughts, and emotions.
4. Now let the client focus on their problem/stress again and explore the body experience associated with it.
5. Support them to pendulate back and forth between the conflict-free state and the stress or pain state.
6. Test, whether the conflict-free image is stronger than the traumatic experience. If not, go back to step 2.
7. Continue to have the client pendulate again between the conflict-free state and the pain state until the symptom clearly diminishes.
8. Consolidate the newly formed pleasant state with breathing techniques (*expansion*) or tapping on the back of the hand.
9. Motivate the client to practice pendulation between the conflict-free experience and the symptom state between therapy sessions.

Therapists can introduce this intervention with the following question:

"When, in your daily life, do you feel most like you would like to feel more often or always?"

If the client does not find anything, the therapist might explain:

> "No matter how unhappy or difficult a life, there are always brief moments that are a bit easier, otherwise survival would not be possible. Take your time. Look for a situation in your daily life that is a bit easier or even pleasant, but at least neutral."

When applying conflict-free experience, step 6 is particularly important, because if the conflict-free experience is not stronger than the symptom and there is no symptom reduction through pendulation, the conflict-free experience is not strong enough or is mixed with something unpleasant. In this case you should look for another stronger everyday experience.

Finding the Conflict-free Zone (Paulsen, 2009)

As mentioned above, there is no consensus on the model of the inner self. However, the notion of such an indestructible core can play an essential role in trauma healing, in consolidating resources, and stabilizing the entire personality.

> "One part of you might feel angry, while another one is quiet. I appreciate both, because both are important for you. Yet I would like to ask both of them to step aside for a moment. Maybe there is also a frightened part and one that is relaxed. I would also like to invite those two to step aside. And maybe one part is sad, and another one is happy. And I'd also like to ask these two to step aside for a moment. Then the therapist continues: How does that feel for you so far? And then: Maybe there is a part that is in pain, and another one that feels good. These two I'd also like to invite to step aside . . . etc. (This is adapted to the specific client.) And then to the client: And what do you notice now?"

Forming an *inner team* (Fritzsche, 2013; Emmerson, 2014) strengthens all ego states and thus the entire personality. This can be done by convoking all relevant parts like in Fritzsche's metaphor of a castle, or by having two or more parts connect and cooperate in a team like in Emmerson's Resource Therapy. However, this does not always have to be an orchestrated gathering of the parts. Often it is more appropriate for therapists to keep the concept of the inner team in the back of their minds, as a possibility to stabilize and strengthen the ego as well as promote cooperation and integration of the ego states. They can then induce the work with the inner team any time and accompany it with their questions, whilst allowing clients to actually shape the process. Here is an example of the work with the "inner team."

Steve, 48, suffers from panic attacks, generalized anxiety, always worrying about his children and his future. He has been in therapy for 1.5 years and already knows some self-regulation techniques. Many of his little scared ego states were able to have corrective experiences and be integrated. Currently, he is troubled by his fear of fear. On a scale of 1 to 10, he rates the intensity at 6–7. Since Steve responded really well to tapping techniques before, the therapist decides to use this instrument for self-regulation. With various Energy Psychology techniques, also regarding self-reproaches (over-energy correction, sentences of self-acceptance, tapping), he can reduce his fear of fear to a 2.

In the following session, Steve reports that the tapping has helped him to calm down, and that he had tapped every day.

In order to stabilize and strengthen the entire personality, the therapist decides to work with the inner team. She asks Steve: I think it would be sensible to convoke the inner team again. What ego states are important today? Who should be on the team today?

Steve, with his eyes closed, says: Courage, Love, Reflexion, and Guilt are already in the conference room. Fear is also in the room. All nervous, she is crawling in the dark, only communicating with the team through Guilt.

Therapist: What is wrong with Fear?
Client: Fear would like to become part of the team, to be accepted and invited to the team.

The therapist invites Steve to introduce Fear to the team and vice versa. During this introduction and while getting to know each other, it becomes obvious that, until now, Fear has been working at night, the other ego states in the daytime. The team is still very careful and reserved towards Fear.

The therapist suggests that Fear also works in the daytime in order to become a full member of the team. This would not have to happen immediately, but could develop slowly.

Therapist: Who could support Fear in switching from the nightshift to the dayshift?
Client: Courage.
Therapist   Courage, are you ready to support Fear in shifting from
(to Courage):   working at night to working in the daytime to be more with the team?

Courage agrees. After this session, Steve's sleeping disorders diminish to a minimum.

Important Factors for the Corrective Experience

The basic foundation of stabilization is not only self-regulation and coregulation and building a trusting therapeutic relationship, but also allowing for a corrective experience of the emerging injured or traumatized states. This confrontational approach aims at a holistic understanding and the overwhelmed state realizing that the threatening situation is over and that it now has the power to change and reshape its inner space. Important factors for the integration of traumatized ego states is their safety and nourishing them retroactively – through ideal parents. The following checklist contains the most important factors for a successful corrective experience.

Checklist: Who is Needed

- Someone who nourishes and is affectionate
- Someone who gives comfort
- Someone who gives security (with babies, this means holding them, cradling, humming, etc.)
- Someone with a good sense of humor who laughs
- Someone who loves unconditionally, with unconditional acceptance
- Someone who protects
- Someone who is wise and offers advice

Bringing Frightened Powerless Ego States into
the Present (in line with Emmerson, 2014)

---

1. The frightened ego state is brought into consciousness by asking the client to name a specific situation in which the undesired feeling occurred (i.e., test anxiety).
2. This specific situation is explored in detail and on all sensory levels by asking the clients to describe the situation in depth, in the present form, as in: What do you see? What do you hear? What clothes are you wearing? Who else is there?
3. When the state is present, it is addressed by the therapist directly and asked its name: What may I call you? If it does not know a name, the therapist suggests one (Powerless? Little One?).
4. Now the therapist finds out about the state's feelings, sensations, and age: Where in your body do you feel powerless now? How large is this sensation? Is it bright or dark? Is there a color? If a client appears to be

young or small: To me, this sounds like a child. If the client says yes: How old does this child feel? If client says no, the therapist continues exploring. The therapist can also ask directly about the age: How old do you feel? With some clients, an intellectual part then steps in, giving the client's current age, so it is worth continuing to enquire and explore in detail.

5. Now the therapist tries to find out where the state is: Powerless, are you in a building or outside? Are you alone or is somebody there? What is happening? Is somebody or something there threatening you?

6. Now the frightened state is empowered until it feels safe: Powerless, this is not happening now, it is over. You are safe here. This is a memory you can now change. You now have the power to do that. If the state is threatened: You can shrink them (the perpetrators) or it (what is threatening), so they are small, and put them further away until you feel safe. You can design your inner space as it is good for you.

7. The therapist now invites the empowered state to express its feelings: They're only memories, and not really here now, so you can look at them and tell them anything you want! You could say: Leave me alone! Or perhaps: You're mean!

8. After everything has been said, the empowered state can decide whether it still wants to keep the threatening figures or what is threatening in its inner space. If not, which is normally the case, the therapist invites the client to remove the threatening figures out of their inner space.[1]

9. If necessary, the inner space is also secured with a magical boundary, and with the help of the client resources are found to accompany the empowered state, and to nourish and protect it retroactively.

10. Finally, the ego state that used to be frightened is now asked about its feelings again: Powerless, how is it now? Are you really sure? And do you understand that it will remain like that from now on? Does the name "Powerless" still fit? No? What name would be better? Cheerful? Then I will call you "Cheerful" from now on, a nice name!

11. If necessary, the therapist can find a resource state together with the client that supports them with the desired behavior in daily life: I would now like to speak to a part that can support you with your exams so that you can approach them with the desired composure. The therapist also speaks to this ego state directly, asking its name and whether it wants to take over the task. The resource state will gladly do that. (*Finding resource*)

12. Next, the therapist asks again about the specific situation: How is it now? It should feel distinctly different for the client.

Nourishing Retroactively, Corrective Experiences

First, a connection to the safe place or a resource is established.

Contact with the injured, frightened or traumatized part is established through the affect bridge, the somatic bridge, or age regression, i.e., the memory of a specific situation.

Now the neediness, condition, distress and urgency of the ego state is determined: What does the injured part need? When the stress becomes too great for the client, the therapist invites them to take the perspective of an observer. The injured ego state can be addressed directly, the therapist convincing it that its experience belongs to the past: This is not happening now, it is a memory! You are now safe here and have the power to change everything so it is good for you and you feel safe. It's over now. What would you like to change? What do you need most right now?

Empowering the frightened ego state in this way must be done before retroactive nourishing.

First, the therapist checks whether the injured ego state wants to leave the traumatic situation and go to a safe place or whether the injured ego state can change its environment, so it becomes safe.

Only when the ego state feels safe does the therapist suggest getting a nourishing protecting being that will take care of it in the future (this can be a person, a resourceful ego state, an animal, an angel, a protagonist from a film or a story, or a mythical creature).

Now the client imagines and feels in detail how this creature takes care of them or protects them, so the ego state rescued from fear and helplessness can connect safely and reliably with this creature.

Retroactive nourishing, the corrective experience, is accompanied, deepened, and reinforced in accordance with the age of the injured ego state, and adapted to its needs.

How does it feel now for the formerly injured ego state? With the sensations of the state, the client's physical resonance is explored, and the therapist also senses into how the protective and nourishing creature is doing. What effect does this experience have on the whole body?

Now the formerly frightened ego state is assured by the therapist that it will always stay like that, that it is not to blame, that it is entitled to this caring and unconditional love and that it is sad that it did not get that a long time ago.

To complete the corrective experience, the therapist checks again whether the formerly traumatized part now has everything it needs and has understood everything.

Then the client is asked to go back to their safe place or to contact a resource, after which they are reoriented in time and space.

Finally, the client is invited to check how they are doing and the resonance in their body including all associated sensations.

Trance for Self-Regulation and Integration through Shifting (Pendulation)/Simultaneity

The following trance promotes self-regulation and integration and was developed by the author according to Kaiser-Rekkas (2009) and Daitch (2007).

Make yourself at home, seating yourself as comfortably as possible in your chair, and contact the floor . . . Now I'd like to invite you to remember a situation in your life where you were totally at peace with yourself . . . in tune with yourself . . . Maybe several situations pop up . . . take your time . . . until one situation crystallizes, where you were completely at peace with yourself . . . Remember the details . . . where you were, what you saw, heard, all the details you need to feel and experience again, what it was like . . . body sensations, thoughts, where in your body do you notice this specifically? . . . Maybe it is everywhere . . . And now, Mrs. X., think of a situation in the last few days if there was one, otherwise a little longer ago, where you felt at odds with yourself . . . And also remember the details you need so you can really feel this state . . . What was it like to be at odds with yourself? Where in your body do you notice this particularly . . .? And maybe, Mrs. X., you can now imagine that the part that can be at peace with itself goes to the part that is at odds with itself and gets in touch with it in a friendly, loving, and accepting way . . . The part that can be at peace with itself goes to the one that is at odds with itself, establishing contact in a friendly . . . loving . . . accepting way, with words, touch . . . maybe also energetically or all of that together . . . just as it feels right for you now. . . it is important that it is supportive . . . that it is affectionate . . . the way you take care of someone you love and who might be in trouble . . .

And now, Mrs. X, I'd like you to imagine that you take both. . . ., Both parts into your heart . . . You can picture that you are holding one part in each hand . . ., and you can allow your hands to slowly make their way to your heart, at their own pace, where you can take them both into your heart . . . Just let your hands do it . . . They know how . . . it must be so both parts reach the heart at their pace, in their own time. Because, strictly speaking, all of that is you . . . Your self from this morning includes both states . . . Sense how that feels, what it is like . . . that both can be in your heart . . . And if you like, Mrs. X, you can imagine, that you are enveloped . . . surrounded by a light, a very special light . . . only for you . . . A light signifying peace, a peaceful light enveloping you . . . giving you security . . . For many people it is blue or the blue of a summer sky in Italy, a color giving peace . . . If that suits you, you can imagine that you are sitting in this light or that the light is flowing through you . . . maybe it is another color, only you know what your light, your light of peace enveloping and flowing through you, looks like . . . And the light gives heat and light . . . you can let it come into every corner of your heart so that your heart is all bright and warm . . . And, as a next step, you might imagine that, with every breath, this warmth and brightness from the heart gradually spreads in your whole chest . . . very good . . . spreading with each breath and from there further on into your entire body . . . the warming, bright light of peace . . . so that your body is gradually filled more and more with this warmth . . . this brightness, the light of peace . . . and maybe, Mrs. X, you can imagine that this light . . . is streaming out of your heart through the soles of your feet . . . so that, with every breath . . . a circle of light is formed around you . . . and maybe you can imagine that this light in your heart is inexhaustible . . . inexhaustible . . . there is always brightness and warmth . . .

And now invite the person you were maybe ten or maybe two years ago, or maybe even a younger person, whatever is right now, into this circle of light . . . and give that person or those people, there might be more than one younger one, the warmth and brightness from your heart so that the younger selves also get warm and bright, warm and bright and peaceful . . . Maybe you would also like to bring in the teenager you once were into the circle of light . . . and give her the light from your heart . . . so that she can feel warm and bright . . . And maybe you would also like to invite a school child into your circle of light that is warming, and bright and peaceful . . . And maybe also the toddler that you were before going to kindergarten . . . And you give her light from your heart . . . And in your peaceful circle of light she is safe with you . . . And maybe, Mrs. X, you would like to imagine the person you will be when you are old . . . and would like to invite that person into your circle of light . . . the one you will be tomorrow . . . Maybe the one from tomorrow having to cope with so much . . . Only you know what is needed now. And maybe there is another self, a state you believe to be really, really needy, or might become very needy . . . Also give this self the warmth and the light from your heart that is now in you. Also envelop her in warmth and light . . .

Finally, Mrs. X, you can confirm for yourself . . . I am full of warmth and compassion for myself . . . and I trust that this ability will always be available to me whenever I want . . .

Take a moment before completing this exercise . . . knowing . . . you can return to this state anytime . . . And when your body or your organism is ready . . . it can breathe deeply, and hand and feet can slowly start moving again . . . maybe your fingers and toes first . . . then your hands and feet . . . allowing the body to stretch so it can wake itself up again . . . tensing the muscles and stretching like a kitten in the sun . . . and waking itself again through a deep breath . . . and then, when your body, your organism is ready . . ., you can slowly open your eyes and come into contact with your environment.

Welcome to the World (in line with Poole Heller, 2017)

Purpose: Many adults suffer from negative or insecure attachment imprints and from feelings of worthlessness, because their parents could not build a safe attachment with them as children. These attachment patterns in the brain can be changed towards more safety, with the effect of feeling safer and better in real relationships as well.

Preparation:

- First read the whole exercise.
- Create a comfortable meditative space where you can be undisturbed and can close your eyes for 15 minutes.
- If you like, switch on quiet, peaceful music in the background.
- Write a list of 3 to 12 people with whom you feel safe, who support and accept you. These people can be real, or they can simply exist in your imagination. Who do you want to be present at your birth?

Exercise:

- Turn on the music and find a comfortable position in your chair.
- Relax and breathe quietly and regularly for a few minutes.
- Imagine that this is now the moment of your birth. You do not have to include your real parents in the image if you do not want to. This is going to be the best birth there can be for you.
- After you have been born, imagine that you are wrapped into a nice, warm cozy blanket. Imagine the first visitor – somebody from your list. What does this person say to you? What are the words of welcome that you hear first? Let them say these words slowly and carefully. Maybe they touch you, hold you, or rock you.
- Take your time – hear every word. Feel each one of them also in your body. Feel the touch and also the support and how you are being held. Let the next person come, and so on. Then place all the visitors in a circle around you. Feel how this group becomes your support group for your life.
- You are also given a gift by the people, and each gift has a specific meaning. Feel the presence of the people around you. Inhale everything.
- You can repeat this exercise as often as you like.

Loving Eyes

"Seeing oneself with loving eyes" (Knipe, 2008) is a very helpful exercise for clients with very early or attachment trauma, for people with complex trauma, and those with dissociative phenomena.

Step 1:

Therapist helps the adult client to be in a good contact with themselves, and to feel safe in the here and now. Only then does the therapist ask the adult to observe the (traumatized) child from back then – with some distance from the child: Sitting here, can the adult of today look at the child from back then?

Step 2:

If clients agree, the therapist says: Look at the child. Notice it. It is only about noticing what feelings and experiences this child has, unconditionally, without judging . . .

Step 3:

Adult clients often have a deprecative, judgmental attitude towards the child. This negative attitude is an unconscious defense and protection reaction – especially when shame is involved. Or it helps to keep up dissociation for pain control.

Therapist asks: What is good about knowing today that you are no longer this child? That it is over? What is good about knowing that you are no longer in this situation, that you are not stupid or weak or dirty or powerless . . .?

After the client has replied, the therapist continues: Think about it. Stay with this realization for a moment.

Usually, the feeling of shame diminishes in favor of compassion for the child and the client reaches the understanding that: This was really in a situation where the child could not do anything. The child didn't have a choice . . . Or: The child couldn't help it. The therapist, in turn, confirms that.

Step 4:

Therapist: When you see the child – can you see its feelings? What facial expression does the child have? Posture?

Step 5:

When a client starts speaking more empathetically about the child, the therapist can continue: If you look at the child, what do you feel in regard to the child?

The client is invited to look at the child from back then "with loving eyes," with love and respect.

Can the child hear you? Is there something that you as an adult can now do for the child, something that would feel helpful? Would you like to tell the child something, explain something?

Take your time for this inner dialogue.

Step 6:

If a client reports that the child is afraid to be seen, criticized, or laughed at, or if they cannot look at the child with loving eyes (yet), the focus should be redirected to the adult self:

If you as an adult look at the child – what is your gaze like? Critical? Judgmental? If the client affirms this, the therapist returns to step 3: Do you think that the child is having a hard time? Or:

If a friend's child or a child you love were in the same situation, could you look with compassion? What is it like then?

Goal: Clients should be able to look at the child with respect and compassion.

Empowering Interventions in Ego State Therapy

Contact with Ego States on a Somatic Level (Phillips, 2016)

1. Identify a resource ego state.
2. Find this state through body sensations, symptoms, feelings, memories, symbols, images, inner dialogue, posture, or movement. Explore the qualities and boundaries of these states in the body.
3. Now observe a state associated with unpleasant feelings, with irritation, hyperactivation, or hypoactivation. Also explore qualities and boundaries here. Beware not to remain here for too long so it does not become too unpleasant for the client: Respect their window of tolerance.
4. Use breathing techniques to connect the two states, or pendulate back and forth between the two.
5. Discover whether there is a conflict between the two states.
6. Explore whether the ego states express themselves through movements.
7. Find out how the two states cooperate and can help each other.

Alternative:

The client thinks of a problem and feels the body sensations associated with it. The therapist explores The therapist explores SIBA-reactions (sensations, imagination, behavior/movement, affects).

If it is suitable, different ego states, or states, are found and explored. This should be limited to three ego states.

The therapist supports the client to understand their role/function/ quality. It is helpful to first look out for differences and then for common ground.

The body is given enough time so the two parts can integrate or help each other.

Circle of Strength (Phillips, 2015)

1. A circle of strength is made of real people who are important for one's life – partner, friends, family members giving safety, mentors, spiritual teachers, or other allies from all phases of life.
2. Who showed up? Everyone who is present gives strengthening supportive messages/energies and all these messages/energies are accepted.
3. Now a reply is given to all these messages/energies of the circle.

The circle of strength can always be invoked, if shame, doubt, or other negative feelings pop up.

Working with Ego States Overwhelmed with Rejection (Emmerson, 2014)

1) With a specific situation, the state suffering from rejection is brought into consciousness.
2) The body sensations, and the feelings associated with it, are explored and, if possible, given a form, by finding inner images, until clients have completely immersed themselves in the original experience.
3) As soon as the state shows itself, it can be addressed directly. The therapist invites it to tell the introject by which it feels rejected its feelings and thoughts directly. (For this, an empty chair is placed across from the client.)
4) The client is then asked to take a seat on the empty chair and to answer as the introject directly and spontaneously. The therapist speaks directly to the introject, which in turn addresses the rejected state directly, thus increasing understanding of the inability of the rejecting introject to love unconditionally.
5) Now the client is invited to return to their chair, and as soon as they sit down the rejected ego state is addressed with its name. The therapist makes sure that it has understood that, like any child, it deserves to be loved unconditionally, but that the introject was not able to. The rejected ego state can now decide whether it wants to keep the introject in its inner space or prefers to send it to another place where it is cared for.
6) Now, the formerly rejected part, still feeling fragile, is supported by a nourishing ego state, to secure protection and care.
7) Again, clients are invited to imagine the specific situation explored at the beginning. If the intervention was successful, this situation should clearly be experienced as being different, with relief or distance.

Unlike Emmerson's procedure, we do not speak of "removal" of the introject, but rather of sending it away from the inner space, yet not from the inner stage.

Negotiations with Retro States (Emmerson, 2014)

This intervention should happen *after* the treatment of the state involved, overwhelmed with fear or rejection, because only then is the Retro State ready to change.

---

1. Through a specific situation where the unwanted behavior pops up the Retro State is contacted.
2. By communicating directly with this state, the therapist can find out how it helped the client: What was its intention? What would have happened if you hadn't sprung into action? Please consider this: The state's intention is good; its *behavior* is unwanted.
3. First you thank the Retro State for having stood up for the client. This appreciation for its *efforts* is important even if the state's behavior has negative consequences. Note that it is not the behavior or the role that's being praised, but the effort, the good intention behind it. And the fact that the state risked being rejected by the other ego states with this strategy can also be acknowledged.
4. Now a name can be found for the Retro State relating to its good intention and not to its behavior: For example, you would not be speaking of the "drinker" but rather of "flight" or "appeaser." The therapist can suggest a name, but the Retro State decides whether it fits.
5. A new alternative role is suggested with which the state can pursue its original intention but in such a way that it is appreciated by the other states and the client. Important: At the time of the intervention, the state is not yet asked whether it wants to take on this new role. First other states or clients are asked whether they would appreciate the Retro State with the new behavior. Retro states can often not imagine taking on a different behavior, and even less being loved by the other states. That is why this step needs sufficient time and care. Therapists might say to the Retro State: I understand that you cannot imagine at this point doing something else or even being liked and appreciated by the other states or by Mr. X. It is much too early for that now, but I do believe that the other states would be happy and would become friends with you.
6. Then the therapist asks one or more other ego states or the client what they would think of the Retro State's new role: Would you be happy if, from now on, Flight would report the first signs of stress and thus help to flee? The states involved should then be invited to tell the Retro State directly that they would like and appreciate it if it changed its behavior.

7. Then the therapist speaks to the Retro State again: Flight, did you hear that? The other states will like you, appreciate you, and be pleased with your new role! And yet you can still live up to your important intention and help Mr. X (the client). Is that okay for you?

The Separation Sieve (Emmerson, 2014)

The separation sieve helps clients with letting go of unpleasant feelings such as guilt and trauma or the connection to an ex-partner.

1. The therapist makes sure that the ego state with the feelings is activated.
2. The therapist checks whether there is truly a readiness to let go.
3. The state is invited to imagine the separation sieve: Imagine something like a magical sieve or a magic filter. I don't know what exactly that looks like, only you know that. Now you can pass through this sieve or filter or whatever you can imagine, and all the heavy, dark, dirty, sticky, unpleasant stuff, everything negative that you no longer want, remains in the sieve as you move through. This is only an experiment. Once you are on the other side, you can always decide whether you want something back. Some people imagine letting themselves fall through the sieve.
4. When you are ready, allow what is light and free, the pure essence of you, to go or fall through the sieve and everything that is dark, heavy, dirty, sticky, everything you no longer want, remains in the sieve. Give me a sign when you have passed through it.
5. How does it feel now? (Usually, much lighter and brighter.)
6. Look back to the sieve and describe what the stuff looks like that got caught. (If nothing remains in the sieve, the therapist can suggest to cleanse it, make it more closely meshed and less permeable. Then the process can be repeated.)
7. Do you want any of it back? (Normally, the response is "No." Otherwise the state should retrieve what was filtered.)
8. What color or what light is strong enough to completely dissolve what remained in the sieve?
9. When you are ready, let the light or color sizzle away all the dark, nasty stuff in the sieve. Zzzzzzzzzzzzzzz! (hissing noise).
   (Sometimes several runs will be necessary for all the unpleasant feelings to be gone.)
10. How do you feel now?

*The Door of Forgiveness (according to
Watkins & Watkins, 1997)*

After induction of a hypnotic trance with a deepening of the trance (i.e., using the stair metaphor – every step leading a little deeper into trance): Now we are at the bottom end of the stairs. In front of us is a long corridor, at the end of which is the Door of Forgiveness. But before you go through the Door of Forgiveness, you might have to go through other doors first, which are situated along both sides of the corridor. Look at the entire corridor and see whether you find any doors. . . . (The therapist waits for a reaction. If the client describes in more detail doors they have seen, continue.) Through which door would you like to go first? Good. Now go to that door and describe to me exactly what that door looks like, even the handle. Have you ever seen this door before? Now that you are standing here, I'd like to invite you to open that door and to tell me what you see. . . . Now enter . . . (When the client has gone through all the doors, it is time for the Door of Forgiveness.) Now go to the end of the corridor, to the Door of Forgiveness. Now that you are standing in front of the Door of Forgiveness, what do you see? . . . When you are ready, open the door. You can now walk through the door and enter the room on your own and experience what is good and necessary for you. You can do that silently or express what is happening. Just give me a sign when you are finished. (After this step, the client is invited to reorient.)

Inner Dialogue with the Help of Chairs (Emmerson, 2014)

The therapist puts an empty chair in front of the client and asks them, or the state overwhelmed with confusion, to imagine that the person or the introject (i.e., Mother) that confuses them or with which they are in conflict, is sitting there.

Therapist: We know that they are not really here, so you can tell them anything you want, you are safe here. Tell them directly!

Once the client or the state has expressed themselves, the therapist asks the client to sit on the empty chair. Just before they take a seat, the therapist calls them by the name of the person or the introject: Mother, have you heard that? How does that feel? The therapists also lets Mother speak directly to the client or the state.

Then the therapist asks the client to return to their own chair. While they are sitting down, they call them by their own name or the name of the state.

This increases the understanding of clients for the introject or the other person, often dissolving rigid patterns or allowing for spontaneous insights.

Organically caused Symptoms (Emmerson, 2014)

The therapist lets the client describe their symptoms in detail and asks them about associated body sensations.

Then they ask this "reporting" state its name and thanks it for "carrying" the pain or the symptom.

Then the therapist asks for a brave, strong, important, and helpful part that can take over the pain by choice so that the reporting state does not have to carry it. The therapist promises the brave ego state that it will be getting appreciation from the other states and from the client for doing so.

The therapist also asks this brave strong part its name and invites it to now take on the symptom or the pain so that the reporting state no longer has to do that, informing the brave part about the possibility of the separation sieve should it be too much for it, and shows it how it works.

Now the reporting part tells the brave one directly how much it appreciates what it is doing, allowing for the latter to reply directly.

Finally, the therapist thanks all the states.

In the next session, the therapist will contact all involved states again and ask them how they are doing.

Psychosomatically Caused Symptoms (Emmerson, 2014)

The therapist has the client describe exactly what the symptom or pain, as well as the associated body sensations, are.

Then therapist asks about emotions and where the client can feel them in the body (usually this is not where the pain is).

After that, the identical procedure is used as with states overwhelmed by fear or rejection described above, so that the corrective experience can happen.

Helpful Tapping Techniques

General Guidelines

Before and after tapping, or rather always when clients are in emotionally stressful or blocking states, it is important that both the therapist and client drink water! The therapist can offer water at the beginning of the session and later invite the client to drink again, making sure that they themselves get enough water.

For the self-regulation of anxiety states and whenever the nervous system is out of balance, crossing limbs or the over-energy correction works wonders. It is an inherent part of the multimodal trauma therapy presented here.

Over-energy Correction

Please find the instructions in Chapter 8, in the section on "Self-regulation through Over-energy Correction".

Resolving Self-reproaches

Self-acceptance with Self-reproaches:

The right hand is placed on the point of self-acceptance over the heart region and moved in a circle, while speaking out loud the following sentences of self-acceptance:

Although I (still) blame myself for _____ ,
I love and accept myself as I am. (The wording can be individualized with the client).

Now you ask yourself whether you were not able or did not want to act differently than how you did. Then you say the following sentence out loud twice, while tapping the nail of your index finger:

And now I forgive myself with all my heart, because I realize that I could/ would not act differently – my word of honor! When saying the last words, you can raise the right hand as with a vow. This brings relief and boosts self-worth (Bohne, 2016).

Resolving Blaming Others

Self-acceptance when Blaming Others:

The right hand is placed on the point of self-acceptance over the heart region and moved in circles while saying out loud the following sentences of self-acceptance:

Although I (still) blame _____ for_____, I love and accept myself the way I am and leave the responsibility for their behavior with them (Bohne, 2016).

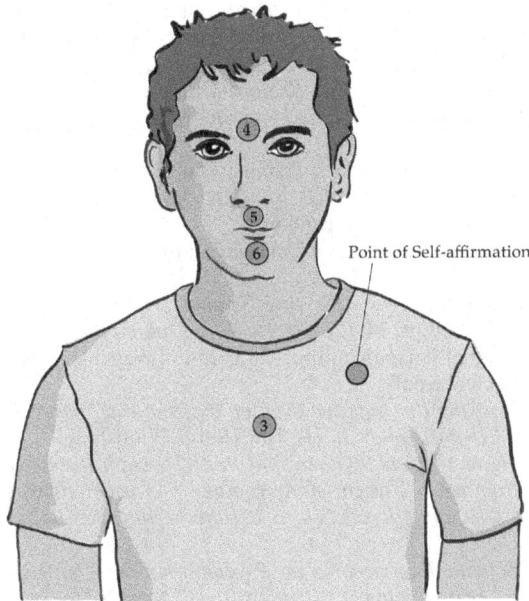

Figure 8.2 Point of self-affirmation and activation points

Note

1 Unlike Emmerson's model, the introject is not removed, but merely sent away from the inner space of the ego-state so that it becomes safe.

References

Bohne, M. (2016): *Klopfen mit PEP. Prozess- und Embodimentfokussierte Psychologie in Therapie und Coaching.* Heidelberg: Carl Auer.

Daitch, C. (2007): *Affect Regulation Toolbox: Practical and Effective Hypnotic Interventions for the Over-Reactive Client.* New York: Norton.

Doidge, N. (2008): *The Brain That Changes Itself. Stories of Personal Triumph from the Frontiers of Brain Science.* Penguin Books Ltd.

Emmerson, G. J. (2014): Resource Therapy. The Complete Guide with Case Examples & Transcripts. Victoria: Old Golden Point.

Frederick, C. a. Phillips, M. (1995): *Healing the Divided Self. Clinical and Ericksonian Hypnotherapy: Clinical and Ericksonian Hypnotherapy for Dissociative Conditions.* W.W. Norton & Company, Inc.

Fritzsche, K. (2013): *Praxis der Ego-State-Therapie.* Heidelberg: Carl-Auer.

Gendlin, E. T. (2003): *Focusing. How to get Direct Access to your Body's Knowledge.* Revised and updated 25th anniversary edition. E-Book. London: Random House.

Kaiser-Rekkas, A. (Ed.) (2009): *Wie man ein Krokodil fängt, ohne es zu verletzen. Innovative Hypnotherapie.* Heidelberg: Carl-Auer, 2., unchanged edition 2013.

Knipe, J. (2008): Loving Eyes. Procedures to Therapeutically Reverse Dissociative Processes while Preserving Emotional Safety. In: C. Forgash & M. Copeley Healing the Heart of Trauma with EMDR and Ego State Therapy. pp. 181–225. New York: Springer.

Levine, P. (2015): *Trauma and Memory: Brain and Body in a Search for the Living Past: A Practical Guide for Understanding and Working with Traumatic Memory.* North Atlantic Books U.S.

Levine, P. (2011): *Somatic Experiencing®.* Training Manual 1st– 3rd year in German. Zurich.

Levine, P. (2010): *In an Unspoken Voice: How the Body Releases Trauma and Restores Goodness.* Berkeley: North Atlantic Books.

Levine, P. (2008): *Healing Trauma: A Pioneering Program for Restoring the Wisdom of Your Body.* Boulder, CO: Sounds True.

Levine, P. (1997): *Waking the Tiger – Healing Trauma.* Berkeley: North Atlantic Books.

Levine, P., Porges, S, & Phillips, M. (2015): *Healing Trauma and Pain Through Polyvagal Science.* E-Book: https://maggiephillipsphd.com/Polyvagal/EBookHealingTraumaPain ThroughPolyvagalScience.pdf

Paulsen, S. (2009): *Looking through the Eyes of Trauma and Dissociation. An Illustrated Guide for EMDR Therapists and Clients.* BookSurge Publishing.

Phillips, M. (2016): *How to Heal Trauma and Pain Through the Body: Somatic Psychotherapy Level 3,* (Seminar in Zurich, 30 September–1 October 2016).

Phillips, M. (2015): *Somatic Approaches to Psychotherapy, Level 2.* Seminar in Zurich, 2–3 October 2015.

Phillips, M. (2014): *Somatic Experiencing for Psychotherapists who Work with Trauma &/or Ego State Therapy, Level 1* (Seminar in Zurich, 16–17 May 2014).

Phillips, M. (2008): *Healing the Trauma-Pain Connection.* (Keynote International Ego State Therapy Congress, 5. Deutsch-nepalesische Ärzte- und Psycholog: innentagung in Kathmandu, Nepal 4–10 May 2008).

Phillips, M. (2007): *Reversing Chronic Pain: A 10-Point All-Natural Plan for Lasting Relief.* North Atlantic Books U.S.

Phillips, M., & C. Frederick (2010): *Empowering the Self through Ego State Therapy.* E-book: http://reversingchronicpain.com/EmpoweringSelfEgoStateTherapy/EST_ebook.pdf

Poole Heller, D. (2017): DARE Program: Dynamic Attachment Re-patterning Experience. Certificate program. www.dianepooleheller.com

Porges, S. W. (1995): Orienting in a Defensive World: Mammalian Modifications of our Evolutionary Heritage. A Polyvagal Theory. *Psychophysiology, 32(4):* 301–318.

Reddemann, L. (2007): *Imagination als heilsame Kraft. Zur Behandlung von Traumafolgen mit ressourcenorientierten Verfahren.* Stuttgart: Klett-Cotta.

Watkins, J., & Watkins, H. (1997)): *Ego States. Theory and Therapy.* W.W. Norton & Company.

Chapter 9

Conclusion

With this book, I hope to orient the reader to healing approaches that help scaffold the possibility of trauma healing. It is by no means an easy journey. Especially with complex and early trauma, clients need time, can only take small steps, and crises must be expected. Often, they cannot achieve complete healing but only a relief of the symptoms. As described in detail in the Introduction, Psychotherapy as an Attachment Workshop, the therapeutic relationship is essential for building trust. In this, clients are just as important as therapists – they need to feel safe in the therapeutic space and always be in control. Thus, they are free to interrupt or break off therapy anytime, which does happen once in a while. The reason is not always the relationship to the therapist or omissions on their part. Sometimes the chemistry is right, but the timing is not. Clients are not always ready (yet) for the pending steps. And, unfortunately, therapy all too often fails because of a lack of financial means. The success of a therapy is always a process shaped by *both* the therapist and the client.

Still, Somatic Ego State Therapy, which includes body knowledge, offers many possibilities to change suffering relatively quickly and with a lasting effect and to strengthen and stabilize people.

The powerful therapy gave me back a part of myself that I had lost.

(46-year-old client)

What helps me with Ego State therapy is that it appeals to my intuition, that the actual reason for the "trauma" does not have to be looked for. My helpers are a part of me, and it does not matter why they came to me back then. I love and appreciate them. The sense of having "released" a new helper helps me to feel myself and my body as a whole, something that I cannot sense very often. It brings quiet and peace, relaxation and freedom.

(31-year-old client)

DOI: 10.4324/9781003460602-10

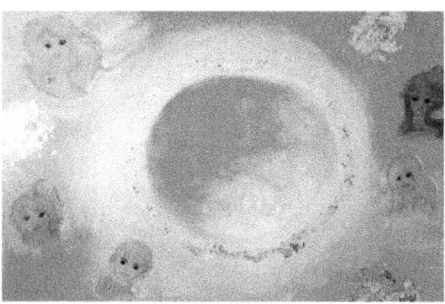

Figure 9.1 Integration – I am whole again! (23-year-old client)

All my parts, united on a wildflower meadow. They all belong to me, finally letting me be whole. My soul is healed. A huge sphere in my heart. Gold, pink, red, orange and yellow. Bright and radiant, warming me and giving me strength, never ever letting me have doubts about myself again. The inner person is finally free and can fly, dance, sing and just be.

(Picture and words from a 23-year-old client, reprinted with permission)

Acknowledgments

A deep thank you goes to all my clients who allowed me to accompany them on their way to wholeness and from whom I have learned so much and am still learning. I hold their courage to face difficult issues in a high regard and am amazed time and again by their creative problem solving and huge self-healing powers. Furthermore, I should like to thank all those who contributed to my book: Maggie Phillips for her mentorship, for her legacy in the field of trauma and pain therapy and for the inspiring Foreword; Woltemade Hartman for connecting a growing Ego State Therapy Community around the world and for the exquisite Preface; Stephen Porges for his corrections; Tobi Goldfus for her precious advice and support in the US; Suzi Tucker for excellent and thorough editing; my daughter Tina Zanotta for helping me untangle format issues; Andrea Bryck for her help and trust; Michelle Graf for her valuable help with writing; Siegfried Joel for his wise and accurate suggestions regarding content and language; Regina Hunter for her coaching and help in structuring the content; and last but not least Grace McDonell of Taylor and Francis for considering my proposal open-mindedly and for making this publication possible.

Besides all my wonderful inspiring trainers of the Milton H. Erickson Society, from whom I learned countless aspects of creative hypnosis, I also thank my Ego State therapy teachers: Maggie Phillips, for allowing me to partake in her rich experiences as an assistant; and also, Claire Frederick, Woltemade Hartman, and Kai Fritzsche, as well as my Somatic Experiencing® teachers: Peter Levine, Kathy Kain, Maggie Kline, and Alé Duarte. I also thank Bernhard Trenkle for organizing many excellent national and international hypnosis congresses, opening up the international perspective and with that also the way to the international Ego State community ESTI for me, as well as the conventions and advanced trainings organized by Woltemade Hartman in such a hospitable way in South Africa.

And last, but not least, I thank my husband Marco for his care, love, and patience.

I hope and wish that the presented principles, proposals, and examples may encourage and inspire as many readers as possible with the occasionally challenging accompaniment of people affected by trauma and give them the confidence of understanding that traumatic experiences can be transformed into life energy and integrated as a resource and become part of the personality.

Index

Locators in **bold** refer to tables and those in *italics* to figures. Alphabetization is word-by-word.